WORKBOOK FOR RADIATION PROTECTION
IN
MEDICAL RADIOGRAPHY

WORKBOOK FOR RADIATION PROTECTION

IN

MEDICAL RADIOGRAPHY

SIXTH EDITION

MARY ALICE STATKIEWICZ SHERER, AS, RT(R), FASRT

3251 Riverport Lane
Maryland Heights, MO 63043

WORKBOOK FOR RADIATION PROTECTION IN MEDICAL RADIOGRAPHY

ISBN: 978-0-323-06608-2

Copyright © 2011, 2006 by Mosby, Inc., an affiliate of Elsevier Inc.

All rights reserved. No part of this publication may be reproduced or transmitted in any form or by any means, electronic or mechanical, including photocopying, recording, or any information storage and retrieval system, without permission in writing from the publisher. Permissions may be sought directly from Elsevier's Rights Department: phone: (+1) 215 239 3804 (US) or (+44) 1865 843830 (UK); fax: (+44) 1865 853333; e-mail: healthpermissions@elsevier.com. You may also complete your request on-line via the Elsevier website at http://www.elsevier.com/permissions.

Notice

Knowledge and best practice in this field are constantly changing. As new research and experience broaden our knowledge, changes in practice, treatment and drug therapy may become necessary or appropriate. Readers are advised to check the most current information provided (i) on procedures featured or (ii) by the manufacturer of each product to be administered, to verify the recommended dose or formula, the method and duration of administration, and contraindications. It is the responsibility of the practitioner, relying on their own experience and knowledge of the patient, to make diagnoses, to determine dosages and the best treatment for each individual patient, and to take all appropriate safety precautions. To the fullest extent of the law, neither the Publisher nor the Author assumes any liability for any injury and/or damage to persons or property arising out of or related to any use of the material contained in this book.

The Publisher

Publisher: Jeanne Olson
Associate Developmental Editor: Amy Whittier
Publishing Services Manager: Catherine Jackson
Senior Project Manager: David Stein
Designer: Paula Catalano

Printed in the United States of America

Last digit is the print number: 9 8 7 6 5 4 3

Working together to grow libraries in developing countries

www.elsevier.com | www.bookaid.org | www.sabre.org

ELSEVIER BOOK AID International Sabre Foundation

Contents

1 Introduction to Radiation Protection, 1

2 Interaction of X-Radiation with Matter, 15

3 Radiation Quantities and Units, 29

4 Radiation Monitoring, 47

5 Overview of Cell Biology, 59

6 Molecular and Cellular Radiation Biology, 71

7 Early Radiation Effects on Organ Systems, 85

8 Late Radiation Effects on Organ Systems, 99

9 Dose Limits for Exposure to Ionizing Radiation, 113

10 Equipment Design for Radiation Protection, 129

11 Management of Patient Radiation Dose during Diagnostic X-Ray Procedures, 145

12 Management of Imaging Personnel Radiation Dose during Diagnostic X-Ray Procedures, 161

13 Radioisotopes and Radiation Protection, 177

Answer Key, 189

1 Introduction to Radiation Protection

Chapter 1 provides an introduction to radiation protection that includes discussion of the use of ionizing radiation in the healing arts, beginning with the discovery of x-rays in 1895. The following topics are covered in this chapter: effective radiation protection, biologic effects, justification and responsibility for imaging procedures, diagnostic efficacy, occupational and nonoccupational dose limits, the as low as reasonably achievable (ALARA) principle, patient protection and patient education, risk versus potential benefit of imaging procedures, and use of background equivalent radiation time (BERT) to inform patients of the amount of radiation they will receive during a specific x-ray procedure. The chapter also discusses types of radiation, the electromagnetic spectrum, ionizing and nonionizing electromagnetic radiation, types of particulate radiation, equivalent dose (EqD) and effective dose (EfD), the biologic damage potential of ionizing radiation, natural and manmade sources of radiation, the accidents at the Three Mile Island–2 (TMI-2) and Chernobyl nuclear power plants, and the use of diagnostic x-ray machines and radiopharmaceuticals in medicine.

CHAPTER HIGHLIGHTS

- Ionizing radiation has both a beneficial and a destructive potential.
- Healthy normal biologic tissue can be injured by ionizing radiation; therefore human beings must be protected against significant and continuous exposure.
- X-rays are a form of ionizing radiation; therefore their use in medicine for the detection of disease and injury requires protective measures.
- Effective radiation protection measures should always be used when diagnostic imaging procedures are performed, in order to safeguard patients, personnel, and the general public.
- Radiation exposure should always be kept ALARA to minimize the probability of any potential damage to people.
- Referring physicians should justify the need for every radiation procedure and accept basic responsibility for the protection of the patient from ionizing radiation.
- The benefits of exposing a patient to ionizing radiation should far outweigh any slight risk of inducing radiogenic cancer or genetic effects after irradiation.
- Radiographers should select the smallest radiation exposure that produces the best radiographic results and should avoid errors that result in repeated radiographic exposures.
- Imaging facilities must have an effective radiation safety program that provides patient protection and education.
- BERT is used to compare the amount of radiation a patient receives from a radiologic procedure with natural background radiation received over a specific period of time.
- Ionizing radiation produces electrically charged particles that can cause biologic damage on molecular, cellular, and organic levels in humans.
- Equivalent dose (EqD) is a radiation quantity used for radiation protection purposes when a person receives exposure from various types of ionizing radiation. This quantity attempts to numerically specify the differences in biologic harm that are produced by different types of radiation. EqD enables the calculation of the effective dose (EfD).
- Effective dose (EfD) takes into account the dose for all types of ionizing radiation to irradiated organs or tissues in the human body. By including specific weighting factors for each body part, such as skin, gonadal tissue and thyroid, EfD takes into account the chance of each of these body parts for developing a radiation-induced cancer (or in the case of the reproductive organs, the risk for genetic damage).
- Both occupational and nonoccupational dose limits are expressed as effective dose.
- Sievert (Sv) and rem are the units of equivalent dose and effective dose.
- Sources of ionizing radiation may be natural or manmade.
  - ☐ Natural sources include radioactive materials in the earth's crust, cosmic rays from the sun and beyond the solar system, internal radiation from radionuclides deposited in humans through natural processes, and terrestrial radiation in the environment.
  - ☐ Manmade sources include consumer products containing radioactive material, air travel, nuclear fuel, atmospheric fallout from nuclear weapons testing, nuclear power plant accidents, and medical radiation from diagnostic x-ray machines and radiopharmaceuticals used in nuclear medicine procedures.

Exercise 1: Crossword Puzzle

Use the clues to complete the crossword puzzle.

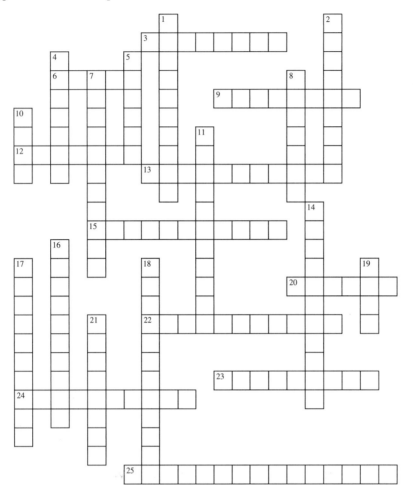

Down

1. Referring to radiation, what EqD and EfD are.
2. Location of nuclear power plant that exploded in 1986 near Kiev in the Ukraine.
4. Radiation produced by human beings (e.g., medical radiation).
5. X-ray examinations that are necessary because of technical error or carelessness.
7. Type of ionizing radiation with energy above 10 eV.
8. Damage to the human body resulting from significant exposure to ionizing radiation.
10. Method that compares the amount of radiation received with natural background radiation received over a given period.
11. Category of ionizing radiation that includes alpha and beta radiation.
14. Most effective tool for early diagnosis of breast cancer.
16. Dose that ultimately may be delivered from a given intake of radionuclide.
17. Effective measures used by radiation workers to safeguard patients, personnel, and the general public.
18. Radiation exposure received by a radiographer during the fulfillment of duties.
19. Possibility of inducing a radiogenic cancer or genetic defect after irradiation.
21. Radiation that produces positively and negatively charged particles when passing through matter.

Across

3. Dark spots that occasionally appear on the sun's surface.
6. Radiation exposure delivered to the whole body over a period of less than a few hours.
9. Electrically neutral components of an atom.
12. Energy that humans can safely control.
13. Type of radiation present in variable amounts in the earth's crust.
15. White blood cells that defend the body against foreign invaders.
20. Radiation of extraterrestrial origin.
22. Radiation exposure that does not benefit a person in terms of diagnostic information obtained for the clinical management of medical needs.
23. Dose level below which individuals would have no chance of sustaining specific biologic damage.
24. Process that is the foundation of the interactions of x-rays with human tissues.
25. Electric and magnetic fields that fluctuate rapidly as they travel through space in the form of a wave.

Exercise 2: Matching

Match the following terms with their definitions or associated phrases.

1. _____ ALARA
2. _____ fallout
3. _____ electromagnetic wave
4. _____ rem
5. _____ BERT
6. _____ radiation protection
7. _____ EqD
8. _____ radionuclide
9. _____ organic damage
10. _____ diagnostic efficacy
11. _____ EfD
12. _____ genetic damage
13. _____ enhanced natural sources
14. _____ biologic effects
15. _____ protons

A. Effective measures employed by radiation workers to safeguard patients, personnel, and the general public from unnecessary exposure to ionizing radiation.
B. The degree to which the diagnostic study accurately reveals the presence or absence of disease in a patient.
C. Traditional unit of measure for the EqD.
D. Damage to living tissue of animals and human beings exposed to radiation.
E. Biologic effects of ionizing radiation or other agents on generations yet unborn.
F. Electric and magnetic fields that fluctuate rapidly as they travel through space, including radio waves, microwaves, visible light, and x-rays.
G. Genetic or somatic changes in a living organism (e.g., mutation, cataracts, and leukemia) caused by excessive cellular damage from exposure to ionizing radiation.
H. Radiation quantity used for radiation protection purposes when a person receives exposure from various types of ionizing radiation. This quantity attempts to numerically specify the differences in biologic harm that are produced by different types of radiation.
I. Radiation quantity that takes into account the dose of all types of ionizing radiation to irradiated organs or tissues in the human body. By including specific weighting factors for each of those parts of the body, such as skin, gonadal tissue, and thyroid, this quantity takes into account the chance of each of those body parts for developing a radiation-induced cancer (or, in the case of the reproductive organs, the risk for genetic damage).
J. SI unit of measure for the EqD.
K. Method for comparing the amount of radiation received from a radiologic procedure with natural background radiation received over a given period.
L. Produces positively and negatively charged particles (ions) when passing through matter.
M. The full range of frequencies and wavelengths of electromagnetic waves.
N. Energy that passes from one location to another.
O. Injury on the cellular level caused by sufficient exposure to ionizing radiation at the molecular level.

16. _____ Sv
17. _____ cellular damage
18. _____ terrestrial radiation
19. _____ radiation
20. _____ beta particle
21. _____ ionizing radiation
22. _____ alpha particle
23. _____ electromagnetic spectrum
24. _____ cosmic rays
25. _____ atomic number

P. Acronym for *as low as reasonably achievable.*
Q. Rays of extraterrestrial origin that result from nuclear interactions that have taken place in the sun and other stars.
R. Long-lived radioactive elements present in variable quantities in the earth's crust; they emit densely ionizing radiations.
S. Contains two protons and two neutrons.
T. Natural sources of ionizing radiation that become increased because of accidental or deliberate human actions, such as mining.
U. Identical to high-speed electrons, except they are emitted from the nuclei of radioactive atoms instead of originating in atomic shells.
V. The number of protons contained within the nucleus of an atom.
W. Positively charged components of an atom.
X. Radiation produced as a consequence of nuclear weapons testing and chemical explosions in nuclear power plants.
Y. An unstable nucleus that emits one or more forms of ionizing radiation to achieve greater stability.

Exercise 3: Multiple Choice

Select the answer that *best* completes the following questions or statements.

1. Which of the following *increases* radiation exposure for both the patient and the radiographer?
   A. Production of optimal quality images with the first exposure
   B. Use of appropriate radiation protection procedures
   C. Repeated radiographic exposures as a result of technical error or carelessness
   D. Limited radiographic examination, as ordered by the radiologist

2. To implement an effective radiation safety program in a facility that provides imaging services, the employer must provide all of the following *except:*
   A. An appropriate environment in which to execute an ALARA program and the necessary resources to support the program
   B. X-ray equipment that can produce only very low kilovoltage and very high milliamperage
   C. A written policy that describes the ALARA program and identifies management's commitment to keeping all radiation exposure as low as reasonably achievable
   D. Periodic exposure audits to determine ways to lower radiation exposure in the workplace

3. According to NCRP Report No. 160, which reflects usage patterns through 2006, radon and thoron account for what percent of natural background radiation exposure?
   A. 15%
   B. 25%
   C. 37%
   D. 55%

4. Occupational and nonoccupational doses will remain well below maximum allowable levels when:
   A. Radiographers and radiologists keep exposure as low as reasonably achievable.
   B. Referring physicians stop ordering imaging procedures.
   C. Orders for imaging procedures are determined only by medical insurance companies.
   D. Patients assume sole responsibility for ordering their imaging procedures.

5. As of 1987, manmade radiation contributed what amount of mSv (mrem) to the annual exposure of the U.S. population?
   A. 0.3 (30)
   B. 0.65 (65)
   C. 1.2 (120)
   D. 3.6 (360)

6. Which of the following places human beings in closer contact with extraterrestrial radiation?
   A. Posteroanterior and lateral digital radiographic images the chest
   B. Deep-sea diving
   C. A flight on a commercial airplane
   D. Visit to a nuclear power plant

7. What do airport surveillance systems; ionization-type smoke detectors; older, luminous dial timepieces; nuclear power plants; and false teeth made of porcelain have in common?
   A. They are all sources of natural background radiation.
   B. They each contribute 0.05 mSv (5 mrem) per year to the equivalent dose received by the global population.
   C. They are not sources of ionizing radiation.
   D. They are all sources of manmade radiation.

8. From which of the following sources do human beings receive the *largest* dose of ionizing radiation?
   A. Radioactive fallout from atomic weapons testing
   B. Medical radiation procedures
   C. Cosmic rays
   D. Area around a nuclear reactor

9. As of 1987, medical radiation exposure from the use of diagnostic x-ray machines and radiopharmaceuticals *collectively* accounted for approximately what amount of the average annual individual effective dose of ionizing radiation?
   A. 0.25 mSv (25 mrem)
   B. 0.54 mSv (54 mrem)
   C. 0.78 mSv (78 mrem)
   D. 0.92 mSv (92 mrem)

10. Of the following groups of people, which group is most likely to experience adverse health effects as a consequence of *substantial* exposure to ionizing radiation?
    A. Employees on duty at TMI-2 at the time of the 1979 nuclear power plant accident
    B. Members of the general population living within 50 miles of the TMI-2 nuclear reactor at the time of the 1979 accident
    C. Members of the general population living near Kiev in the former Soviet Union at the time of the 1986 accident at the Chernobyl nuclear power plant
    D. News reporters visiting the former Soviet Union 10 years after the 1986 Chernobyl accident

11. Which of the following is a radiation quantity used for radiation protection purposes that attempts to numerically specify the differences in biologic harm that is produced by different types of radiation?
    A. Absorbed dose
    B. Background equivalent radiation time
    C. Equivalent dose
    D. Exposure

12. A 3-year pilot research project was launched in the Republic of Belarus in 1996, in the aftermath of the Chernobyl nuclear accident, to empower local citizens in making their own decisions regarding reconstruction of their overall quality of life; this project was known as the:
    A. ALARA Program
    B. Belarus Health Impact Study
    C. Chernobyl Rehabilitation Taskforce
    D. ETHOS Project

13. Any radiation exposure that *does not* benefit a person in terms of diagnostic information obtained for the clinical management of medical needs or that *does not* enhance the quality of a radiologic examination is called:
    A. Artificial radiation
    B. Enhanced natural background radiation
    C. Terrestrial radiation
    D. Unnecessary radiation

14. The amount of radiation a patient receives may be indicated in terms of:
    1. Entrance skin exposure
    2. Bone marrow dose
    3. Gonadal dose
    A. 1 and 2 only
    B. 1 and 3 only
    C. 2 and 3 only
    D. 1, 2, and 3

15. When an imaging procedure is justified in terms of medical necessity, diagnostic efficacy is achieved when optimal-quality images, revealing the presence or absence of disease, are obtained with:
    A. Maximal radiation exposure
    B. Minimal radiation exposure
    C. Scattered radiation exposure
    D. Secondary radiation exposure

16. Ultraviolet radiation below 10 eV, visible light, infrared rays, microwaves, and radio waves are considered to be nonionizing because they:
    A. Have sufficient kinetic energy to eject electrons from atoms
    B. Do not have sufficient kinetic energy to eject electrons from atoms
    C. Have sufficient potential energy to eject electrons from atoms
    D. Do not have sufficient potential energy to eject electrons from atoms

17. Which of the following is a naturally occurring process by which instability of the nucleus is relieved through various types of nuclear spontaneous emissions?
    A. Electromagnetic radiation
    B. Electromagnetic ionization
    C. Radioactive decay
    D. Radioactive fallout

18. Effective radiation protection measures take into consideration:
    1. Both human and environmental physical determinants
    2. Technical elements
    3. Procedural factors
    A. 1 and 2 only
    B. 1 and 3 only
    C. 2 and 3 only
    D. 1, 2, and 3

19. Radioactive elements in the earth's crust and in the human body may be classified as:
    A. Enhanced natural sources of ionizing radiation
    B. Enhanced manmade sources of ionizing radiation
    C. Natural sources of ionizing radiation
    D. Unnatural sources of ionizing radiation

20. Medical radiation procedures account for:
    A. The largest dose of ionizing radiation received by human beings
    B. The second largest dose of ionizing radiation received by human beings
    C. The smallest dose of ionizing radiation received by human beings
    D. Negligible doses of ionizing radiation received by human beings

21. Which of the following commonly used building materials contain(s) radon?
    A. Bricks
    B. Concrete
    C. Gypsum wallboard
    D. All of the above

22. The United States performed above-ground nuclear weapons tests before 1963. During the _____ _____, an atomic cloud was created by a 37-kiloton testing device that was exploded from a balloon at the Nevada test site on June 24, 1957. The top of the atomic cloud, which contained manmade ionizing radiation, ascended approximately 43,000 feet.
    A. Bikini Test
    B. Manhattan Project
    C. Priscilla Test
    D. Rongelap Project

23. The most effective tool(s) for diagnosing breast cancer continue to be:
    A. PA and lateral chest x-ray examinations
    B. Clinical breast self-examination
    C. Clinical breast examination by a physician
    D. Mammography

24. The millisievert (mSv), a subunit of the sievert, is equal to:
    A. $1/10{,}000$ of a sievert
    B. $1/1000$ of a sievert
    C. $1/100$ of a sievert
    D. $1/10$ of a sievert

25. Repetition of a radiographic exposure because of poor patient positioning results in:
    A. No significant change in total radiation exposure to the patient or the radiographer
    B. A slight decrease in total radiation exposure to the patient and the radiographer
    C. An increase in total radiation exposure to the patient and the radiographer
    D. A significant decrease in total radiation exposure to the patient and the radiographer

Exercise 4: True or False

Circle *T* if the statement is true; circle *F* if the statement is false.

1. T F The number of protons in the nucleus of an atom constitutes the atomic number, or "Z".
2. T F The sievert (Sv) is the SI unit of EqD.
3. T F Porcelain used for making dentures is a common example of a consumer product that contains radioactive material.
4. T F A threshold exists for radiation-induced malignant disease.
5. T F BERT is based on an annual U.S. population exposure of approximately 1 mSv per year (approximately 100 mrem per year).
6. T F Radio waves, microwaves, visible light, and x-rays are forms of electromagnetic waves.
7. T F Particulate radiations do not vary in their ability to penetrate matter.
8. T F EfD enables the calculation of the EqD.
9. T F Human beings are not continuously exposed to sources of ionizing radiation.
10. T F A significantly higher number of leukemia cases has been seen in Russian liquidators who worked at the Chernobyl power station complex in 1986 and 1987.
11. T F Atmospheric nuclear testing has escalated since 1980.
12. T F Color television monitors in use today produce substantial radiation exposure for the general public.
13. T F Most radiation-induced cancers have a latent period of 15 years or longer.
14. T F Sources of ionizing radiation may be natural or manmade.
15. T F If emitted from a radioisotope deposited in the body (e.g., in the lungs), alpha particles cannot be absorbed in epithelial tissue and therefore are not damaging to that tissue.
16. T F As of 1987, the average U.S. inhabitant received an equivalent dose of approximately 0.5 mSv (50 mrem) per year from extraterrestrial radiation.
17. T F In the 1987 total, the radon, cosmic ray radiations, and terrestrial and internally deposited radionuclides that comprise the natural background radiation in the United States resulted in an estimated average annual individual equivalent dose of approximately 2.95 mSv (295 mrem).

18. T F Wavelength is the physical distance between successive maximum values of electric and magnetic fields.

19. T F An electron has approximately the same mass as a proton.

20. T F Changes in white blood cell count are a classic example of molecular damage caused by significant exposure to ionizing radiation.

21. T F Some people are exposed to a wide variety of sources of ionizing radiation, whereas others are exposed to a limited number.

22. T F Nonsmokers exposed to high radon levels have a higher risk of lung cancer than do smokers.

23. T F The solar contribution to the cosmic ray background decreases during periods of high sunspot activity.

24. T F Diagnostic efficacy is a vital part of radiation protection in the healing arts.

25. T F When radiographers use their intelligence and knowledge to answer a patient's questions about the risk of radiation exposure honestly, they can do much to alleviate the patient's apprehension and fears during a routine radiologic examination.

Exercise 5: Fill in the Blank

Using the following Word Bank, fill in the blanks with the word or words that best complete the statements.

0.0116	dose rates	radiation dose
1.16	energy	radionuclides (may be used two times)
40	equivalent dose	
600	Ethos Project	radiopharmaceuticals
60,000	far outweigh	radon
ALARA	frequencies	responsibility
beneficial	greatest	risk
benefits	higher	safe operation
BERT	justify	terrestrial
biologic effects	latent period	thyroid
comparison	lowest	wavelengths
cosmic	lung	wave-particle duality
destructive	molten	x-ray machines

1. The actual _____ _____ to the global population from atmospheric fallout from nuclear weapons testing is not received all at once. It is instead delivered over a period of years at changing _____ _____.

2. Most radiation-induced cancers have a _____ _____ of 15 years or longer.

3. The aim of the _____ _____ was to rebuild acceptable living conditions for local citizens in contaminated territories in the Ukraine region of Russia by actively involving them in the reconstruction process.

4. When ionizing radiation is used to obtain a mammogram for the welfare of a patient, the directly realized _____ of the exposure to this radiant energy _____ _____ any slight _____ of inducing a radiogenic malignancy or any genetic defect.

5. In medicine, when radiation safety principles are applied correctly during imaging procedures, the _____ deposited in living tissue by radiation can be limited, thereby reducing the potential for _____ _____.

6. The quantity of _____ radiation present in any area depends on the composition of the soil or rocks in that geographic area.

7. _____ radiation consists predominantly of high-energy protons.

8. The tissues of the human body contain many naturally existing _____, which have been ingested in minute quantities from various foods or inhaled as particles in the air.

9. If a person spends 10 hours flying aboard a commercial aircraft during a period of normal sunspot activity, that individual receives a radiation _____ _____ that is about equal to the dose received from one chest x-ray examination.

10. Medical radiation exposure results from the use of diagnostic _____ _____ and _____ in medicine.

11. Radiologic technologists and radiologists are educated in the _____ _____ of radiation-producing imaging equipment.

12. Electromagnetic radiation appears to have a dual nature, referred to as _____ _____.

13. The _____ concept should serve as a guide for the selection of technical radiographic and fluoroscopic exposure factors for all patient imaging procedures.

14. _____ does not imply radiation risk; it is simply a means for _____.

15. The Environmental Protection Agency (EPA) considers _____ to be the second leading cause of _____ cancer in the United States.

16. _____ in the soil and air add to the human radiation dose burden.

17. The intensity of cosmic rays varies with altitude relative to the earth's surface. The _____ intensity occurs at high altitudes, and the _____ intensity occurs at sea level.

18. Artificial teeth made in the United States are estimated to give the tissues of the oral cavity an average dose of _____ mSv/yr (_____ mrem/yr).

19. As of 1987, when spread over the inhabitants of the United States, fallout from nuclear weapons tests and other environmental sources contributed less than _____ mSv (_____ mrem) annually to the equivalent dose of each person.

20. _____ cancer continues to be the main adverse health effect of the 1986 accident at the Chernobyl nuclear power plant.

21. Referring physicians should _____ the need for every radiation procedure and accept the basic _____ for protecting the patient from ionizing radiation.

22. Ionizing radiation has both a _____ and a _____ potential.

23. During the accident at the TMI-2 nuclear power plant in March, 1979, the U.S. Department of Energy estimated that about _____% of the material in the TMI-2 nuclear reactor core reached a _____ state.

24. In cooler months, when homes and buildings are tightly closed, radon levels are usually _____.

25. The full range of _____ and _____ of electromagnetic waves is known as the *electromagnetic spectrum*.

Exercise 6: Labeling

Label the following illustrations and table.

A. X-ray tube.

B. Percentage contribution of each natural and manmade radiation source to the total collective effective dose for the population of the United States, 2006.

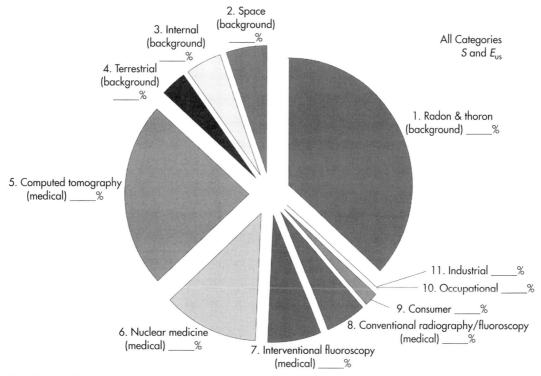

From National Council on Radiation Protection and Measurements (NCRP): *Ionizing radiation exposure of the population of the United States,* Report No. 160, Bethesda, Md, 2009, NRCP.

C. Radiation equivalent dose and subsequent biologic effects of acute whole body exposure*

Radiation Equivalent Dose (EqD)	Subsequent Biologic Effect
1. _____ Sv (_____ rem)	Blood changes (e.g., measurable hematologic depression, decreases in the number of lymphocytes present in the circulating blood)
2. _____ Sv (_____ rem)	Nausea, diarrhea
3. _____ Sv (_____ rem)	Erythema (diffuse redness over an area of skin after irradiation)
4. _____ Sv (_____ rem)	If dose is to gonads, temporary sterility
5. _____ Sv (_____ rem)	50% chance of death; lethal dose for 50% of population over 30 days (LD 50/30)
6. _____ Sv (_____ rem)	Death

Modified from *Radiologic health,* unit 4, slide 17, Denver, Multi-Media Publishing (slide program).
*Radiation exposures are delivered to the entire body over a time period of less than a few hours.

Exercise 7: Short Answer

Answer the following questions by providing a short answer.

1. How can humans safely control the use of radiant energy?

_____

_____

2. How can radiologic technologists reduce radiation exposure to patients and to themselves?

3. How does ionizing radiation damage biologic tissue?

4. What is the basis of the concept of radiation dose?

5. Describe what can happen to a living organism if excessive cellular damage occurs as a consequence of radiation exposure.

6. What is the origin of cosmic radiation? From what does it result?

7. Name four radionuclides found in small quantities in the human body.

8. Why is it impossible to estimate accurately the total annual equivalent dose from fallout?

9. How is risk weighed against benefit in medical radiography?

10. Why does the patient dose for each x-ray examination vary from one health care facility to another?

11. List six consequences of ionization in human cells.

12. What actually produces the sensation of heat or the chemical changes that cause suntan and sunburn?

13. What subunit of the rem is equal to $\frac{1}{1000}$ of a rem?

14. List six sources of manmade, or artificial, ionizing radiation.

15. List three advantages of using the BERT method to compare the amount of radiation received with the natural background radiation received over a given period.

16. What disease continues to be the main adverse health effect of the 1986 accident at the Chernobyl nuclear power plant?

17. List three ways to indicate the amount of radiation received by a patient.

18. What radiation quantity enables the calculation of the effective dose?

19. What is kinetic energy?

20. In terms of ability to penetrate biologic matter, how do alpha particles compare with beta particles? Why are alpha particles considered virtually harmless as an external source of radiation?

Exercise 8: General Discussion or Opinion Questions

The following questions are intended to allow students to express their knowledge and understanding of subject matter or to present a personal opinion on a specific topic. The questions may be used to stimulate class discussion. Because answers to these questions may vary, determination of an answer's acceptability is left to the discretion of the course instructor.

1. Since the 1979 TMI-2 nuclear power plant accident, what detectable effects have been observed in the population living in the community near the plant? What is the current status of TMI-2, and what will eventually happen to this power plant?

2. What mental and adverse physical health effects have been attributed to the 1986 disaster at the Chernobyl nuclear power plant from the time of the accident to the present time? Discuss the consequences of this accident for plant workers, the exposed population, and the remaining global population since the time of the accident. How are the Soviets planning to replace the sarcophagus that covers the remains of the reactor 4 building?

3. Discuss the significance of the ETHOS Project, and explain the value of this program to the community in the Republic of Belarus.

4. How can a radiographer maintain radiation exposure ALARA on a daily basis in a clinical setting?

5. Using the information in Table 1-2 in the text, compare the use, frequency, wavelength, and energy of the radiations that make up the electromagnetic spectrum.

6. Describe the value of patient education with regard to radiation procedures and radiation safety.

7. Discuss the importance of diagnostic efficacy as it relates to medical x-ray procedures and radiation safety for the patient.

8. Discuss the responsibility of the employer in a health care facility for maintaining the ALARA concept in the workplace.

9. Applying the concept of BERT, explain how a radiographer might respond to a patient who asks how much radiation he or she will receive from a routine x-ray series of the lumbar spine.

10. Describe the health impact of radon exposure for humans.

POST-TEST

The student should take this test after reading Chapter 1, finishing all accompanying textbook and workbook exercises, and completing any additional activities required by the course instructor. The student should complete the post-test with a score of 90% or higher before advancing to the next chapter. (Each of the following 20 questions or blanks is worth 5 points.) Score = _____ %

1. Define the term *radiation protection.*

2. What term (and acronym) is used to express the concept of keeping radiation exposure to a level that minimizes the potential for damage to human tissue?

3. Who should justify the need for every radiation procedure and accept basic responsibility for protecting the patient from nonuseful radiation exposure?

4. The benefits of exposing patients to ionizing radiation should far outweigh any slight _____ of induction of radiogenic cancer or genetic defects.

5. What must imaging facilities have that provides for patient protection and patient education?

6. What does ionizing radiation produce that can cause biologic damage on the molecular, cellular, and organic levels in humans?

7. Both occupational and nonoccupational dose limits are expressed as _____ dose.

8. What are the SI unit and the traditional unit of measure for EqD and EfD?

9. Which of the following radiation quantities takes into account the dose for all types of ionizing radiation to irradiated organs or tissues in the body by including specific weighting factors for each body part of concern and taking into account the chance of these parts for developing a radiation-induced malignancy (or, in the case of the reproductive organs, the risk of genetic damage)?
   A. Absorbed dose
   B. Effective dose
   C. Equivalent dose
   D. Exposure

10. Any radiation exposure that does not benefit a person in terms of diagnostic information obtained for the clinical management of medical needs or that does not enhance the quality of a radiologic examination is called:
    A. Enhanced natural background radiation
    B. Environmental radiation
    C. Manmade radiation
    D. Unnecessary radiation

11. Entrance skin exposure (ESE), bone marrow dose, and gonadal dose may be used to indicate:

12. What is the term used for the full range of frequencies and wavelengths of electromagnetic waves?

13. The radioactive elements in the earth's crust and in the human body are considered what type of sources of ionizing radiation?

14. What method can a radiographer use to compare the amount of radiation received during a routine radiographic procedure with natural background radiation received over a given period?

15. The EPA considers the second leading cause of lung cancer in the United States to be:
    A. Diagnostic x-rays
    B. Normal exposure to natural background radiation
    C. Radon
    D. Cosmic rays

16. Which of the following is a consumer product that contains radioactive material?
    1. Porcelain used to make dentures
    2. Airport surveillance systems
    3. Video display terminals that use cathode ray tubes
    A. 1 and 2 only
    B. 1 and 3 only
    C. 2 and 3 only
    D. 1, 2, and 3

17. Are alpha particles more harmful as an external source of radiation or as an internal source of radiation?
    _____

18. Radiographers should select the smallest radiation exposure that produces the best radiographic results and should avoid errors that result in _____ radiographic exposures.

19. What disease continues to be the main adverse health effect of the 1986 accident at the Chernobyl nuclear power plant?
    _____

20. Radiation damage to generations yet unborn defines _____.

2 Interaction of X-Radiation with Matter

Chapter 2 covers the basic concepts of physics that relate to radiation absorption and scatter. The processes of interaction between radiation and matter are emphasized to provide the background that allows radiographers to select the optimal technical exposure factors, such as the peak kilovoltage (kVp) and the milliampere-seconds (mAs). Selection of the appropriate techniques can minimize the radiation dose to the patient and produce optimal-quality images.

CHAPTER HIGHLIGHTS

- Biologic damage in the patient may result from absorption of x-ray energy.
- Variations in the x-ray absorption properties of various body structures make radiographic imaging of human anatomy possible.
- Attenuation results when, through the process of absorption and scatter, the intensity of the primary photons in an x-ray beam decrease as it passes through matter.
- Scattered radiation can result in decreased contrast of the image by adding additional, undesirable gray densities (radiographic fog) or, in fluoroscopy, Compton scattered photons may expose personnel who are present in the room to scattered radiation.
- The amount of energy absorbed by the patient per unit mass is called the *absorbed dose*.
- Two interactions of x-radiation are important in diagnostic radiology: photoelectric absorption and Compton scattering. The photoelectric effect is the basis of radiographic imaging, whereas the Compton effect is its bane.
- For each radiographic procedure, an optimal kVp and mAs combination exists that minimizes the dose to the patient and produces an acceptable image.
  - Within the energy range of diagnostic radiology that includes mammography (23 to 150 kVp), when kVp is decreased, the number of photoelectric interactions increases and the number of Compton interactions decreases; however, the patient absorbs more energy and therefore patient dose increases.
  - When kVp is increased, the patient receives a lower dose, but image quality may be compromised.
  - kVp selection is usually based on the type of procedure and body part to be imaged.
- Radiographers must balance other variables, such as type of image receptor used, patient thickness, and degree of muscle tissue, to arrive at technical exposure factors that will provide an acceptable image yet stay within the standards of radiation protection.
- Coherent scattering is most likely to occur below 10 keV; pair production and photodisintegration occur far above the range of diagnostic radiology.

Exercise 1: Crossword Puzzle

Use the clues to complete the crossword puzzle.

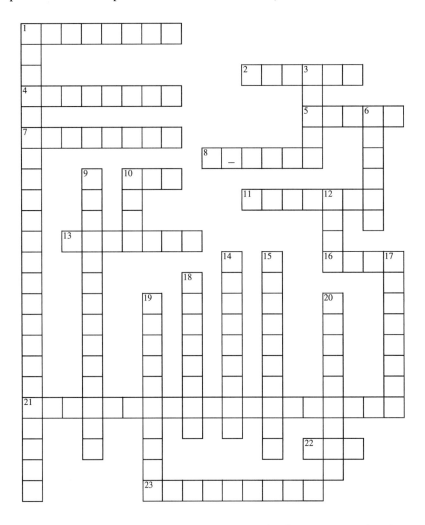

Down

1. Most important mode of interaction between photons and the atoms of the patient's body for producing useful patient images.
3. Type of window in the x-ray tube that permits passage of all but the lowest energy components of the x-ray beam.
6. Type of transmission that occurs when some x-ray photons traverse a patient without interacting.
9. Radiation released as a result of a photoelectric interaction between an x-ray photon and an atom.
10. Type of radiographic image receptor.
12. Seconds during which the x-ray tube is activated.
14. Unit of measure meaning thousands of volts.
15. Type of scattered radiation that degrades the appearance of a completed radiographic image by blurring the sharp outlines of dense structures.
17. Metal with a high melting point and high atomic number from which the target of an x-ray tube is made.
18. Type of damage in the patient that may result from the absorption of x-rays.
19. Another name for coherent scattering.
20. Type of atomic number that is a composite Z number for many different chemical elements composing a material.

Across

1. Form of antimatter.
2. A common method devised to limit the effects of indirectly transmitted x-ray photons.
4. Scattering that occurs when a low-energy photon interacts with one or more free (i.e., unbound) electrons.
5. Target of an x-ray tube.
7. Person responsible for the theory mathematically expressed as $E = mc^2$.
8. Radiation that has neither mass nor electric charge and that travels at the speed of light.
10. Undesirable additional density on a completed radiographic image that can be caused by scattered radiation.
11. Type of energy an x-ray photon possesses.
13. Radiation that emerges directly from the x-ray tube collimator and moves without deflection toward a wall, door, viewing window, and so on.
16. All of the x-ray photons that reach the image receptor.
21. Process of interaction of x-rays with matter that does not occur within the range of diagnostic radiology.
22. Controls the quality, or penetrating power, of the photons in the x-ray beam.
23. What happens to patient dose when kVp increases.

Exercise 2: Matching

Match the following terms with their definitions or associated phrases.

1. _____ absorption
2. _____ permanent inherent filtration
3. _____ photoelectric absorption
4. _____ fluorescent yield
5. _____ mAs
6. _____ kVp
7. _____ deuteron
8. _____ Compton scattering
9. _____ effective atomic number (Z_{eff})
10. _____ aluminum
11. _____ positron
12. _____ radiographic fog
13. _____ attenuation
14. _____ radiographic density
15. _____ photoelectron
16. _____ tungsten rhenium
17. _____ pair production
18. _____ 13.8
19. _____ annihilation radiation

A. Reduction in the number of photons in the x-ray beam through absorption and scatter as the beam passes through the patient in its path
B. Effective atomic number of compact bone
C. Interaction of an x-ray photon with a loosely bound outer-shell electron of an atom
D. Product of electron tube current and the time (in seconds) the x-ray tube is activated
E. Effective atomic number of soft tissue
F. Metal alloy of which the anode of an x-ray tube can be made
G. Transference of electromagnetic energy to the atoms of the patient's biologic material
H. Byproduct of photoelectric interaction
I. Undesirable, additional density on a completed radiographic image that can be caused by scattered radiation
J. Proton–neutron combination
K. Interaction between an x-ray photon and an inner-shell electron of an atom
L. Metal that hardens the x-ray beam by removing low-energy components
M. The highest energy level of photons in the x-ray beam
N. Positively charged electron
O. Combination of the x-ray tube glass wall and the added aluminum placed in the collimator
P. Refers to the number of x-rays emitted per inner-shell vacancy
Q. A composite Z number for many different chemical elements comprising a material
R. The degree of overall blackening on a radiographic image that has been completed
S. Interaction in which the energy of the incoming photon is transformed into two new particles, a negatron and a positron

20. _____ $E = mc^2$
21. _____ 7.4
22. _____ absorbed dose
23. _____ x-ray photons
24. _____ negative contrast media
25. _____ image formation radiation

T. Radiation in the form of two oppositely moving 511-keV photons generated as the result of mutual annihilation of matter and antimatter
U. Mathematical expression of Einstein's theory of relativity
V. The amount of energy absorbed by the patient per unit mass
W. All of the x-ray photons that reach their destination (the image receptor) after passing through the patient being radiographed
X. Agents that result in areas of increased density on a completed image
Y. Particles associated with electromagnetic radiation that have neither mass nor charge and that travel at the speed of light

Exercise 3: Multiple Choice

Select the answer that *best* completes the following questions or statements.

1. When a technical exposure factor of 100 kVp is selected, which of the following occurs?
   A. The energy of the highest energy photon in the x-ray beam is 33 keV.
   B. The electrons are accelerated from the cathode to the anode with an energy of 33 keV.
   C. The energy of the average photon in the x-ray beam is about 100 keV.
   D. The energy of the average photon in the x-ray beam is about 33 keV.

2. The passage of x-ray photons through a patient *without* interaction is called:
   A. Absorption
   B. Attenuation
   C. Scattering
   D. Direct transmission

3. In which of the following x-ray interactions with matter is the energy of the incident photon *completely* absorbed?
   A. Compton
   B. Photoelectric
   C. Incoherent
   D. Rayleigh

4. What is the result of coherent scattering?
   A. Usually just a small angle change in the direction of the incident photon
   B. Transfer of all energy of the incident x-ray photon to the atoms of the irradiated object
   C. Production of a negatron and a positron
   D. Transfer of only some of the energy of the incident x-ray photon to the atoms of the irradiated object

5. A technical exposure factor of 100 kVp means that the electrons bombarding the anode of the x-ray tube have a *maximum* energy of:
   A. 1000 electron volts (eV), or 1 keV
   B. 10,000 eV, or 10 keV
   C. 100,000 eV, or 100 keV
   D. 1,000,000 eV, or 1000 keV

6. A Compton-scattered electron:
   A. Annihilates another electron
   B. Is absorbed within a few microns of the site of the original Compton interaction
   C. Causes pair production
   D. Engages in the process of photodisintegration

7. Most scattered radiation produced during radiographic procedures is the *direct* result of which of the following?
   A. Photoelectric absorption
   B. Nuclear decay
   C. Image-formation electrons
   D. Compton interactions

8. A reduction in the number of primary photons in the x-ray beam through absorption and scatter as the beam passes through the patient in its path defines:
   A. Annihilation
   B. Attenuation
   C. Photodisintegration
   D. Radiographic fog

9. *Before* interacting with matter, an incoming x-ray photon may be referred to as which of the following?
   A. Attenuated photon
   B. Primary photon
   C. Ionized photon
   D. Scattered photon

10. Within the energy range of diagnostic radiology that includes mammography (23 to 150 kVp), when kVp is *decreased,* the patient dose:
    A. Decreases
    B. Increases
    C. Remains the same
    D. Doubles

11. Which of the following statements *best* describes mass density?
    A. It is the number of electrons per gram of tissue.
    B. It is the same as radiographic density.
    C. It relates the way the effective atomic number of biologic tissues influences absorption.
    D. It is measured in grams per cubic centimeter.

12. Of the following interactions between x-radiation and matter, which *does not* occur in the range of diagnostic radiology?
    1. Photoelectric absorption
    2. Pair production
    3. Photodisintegration
    A. 1 and 2 only
    B. 1 and 3 only
    C. 2 and 3 only
    D. 1, 2, and 3

13. For a diagnostic radiologic examination, the selection of technical exposure factors using an *optimal* kVp and mAs combination:
    A. Produces an x-ray image of acceptable quality but increases patient dose
    B. Produces an x-ray image of acceptable quality while minimizing patient dose
    C. Produces an x-ray image of acceptable quality without affecting patient dose
    D. Affects neither the quality of the completed radiographic image nor patient dose

14. The quality, or penetrating power, of an x-ray beam is controlled by:
    A. The absorption characteristics of the patient being radiographed
    B. Fluorescent yield
    C. mAs
    D. kVp

15. Small-angle scatter:
    A. Degrades the appearance of a completed radiographic image by blurring the sharp outlines of dense objects
    B. Enhances the appearance of a completed radiographic image by clearly delineating the sharp outlines of dense objects
    C. Affects the appearance of a completed radiographic image only when contrast medium is used for visualization of a tissue or structure
    D. Occurs only in therapeutic radiologic ranges

16. Within the energy range of diagnostic radiology, as absorption of electromagnetic energy in biologic tissue increases, the potential for biologic damage:
    A. Decreases slightly
    B. Decreases significantly
    C. Increases
    D. Remains the same

17. Which of the following terms are synonymous?
    1. Coherent scattering
    2. Classical scattering
    3. Unmodified scattering
    A. 1 and 2 only
    B. 1 and 3 only
    C. 2 and 3 only
    D. 1, 2, and 3

18. Noninteracting and small-angle scattered photons comprise:
    A. Absorbed photons
    B. Attenuated photons
    C. Exit, or image formation, radiation
    D. Compton scatter

19. *Direct transmission* means that x-ray photons:
    A. Are absorbed in biologic tissue on interaction
    B. Are scattered on interaction with biologic tissue
    C. Pass through biologic tissue without interaction
    D. Pass through biologic tissue with some interaction

20. Which of the following has the same mass and magnitude of charge as a negatron?
    A. Deuteron
    B. Neutron
    C. Positron
    D. Proton

21. Which of the following interactions between x-radiation and matter *does not* occur within the range of diagnostic radiology?
    A. Coherent scattering
    B. Compton scattering
    C. Photoelectric absorption
    D. Pair production

22. kVp controls:
    A. Absorption characteristics of the body part being radiographed
    B. Fluorescent yield
    C. Random interaction of x-ray photons with the image receptor
    D. Quality, or penetrating power, of the photons in the x-ray beam

23. *Primary radiation* is synonymous with:
    A. Direct radiation
    B. Compton scatter
    C. Elastic scatter
    D. Rayleigh radiation

24. Which of the following are radiographic image receptors?
    1. Radiographic grid
    2. Digital radiography receptor
    3. Phosphor plate
    4. Radiographic film
    A. 1 and 2 only
    B. 1 and 4 only
    C. 2, 3, and 4 only
    D. 1, 2, 3, and 4

25. The process most responsible for the contrast between bone and soft tissue in a diagnostic radiographic image is:
    A. Coherent scattering
    B. Compton scattering
    C. Photoelectric absorption
    D. Photodisintegration

Exercise 4: True or False

Circle *T* if the statement listed below is true; circle *F* if the statement is false.

1. T F The radiographer also benefits when patient dose is minimal because less radiation is scattered from the patient.
2. T F The optimal x-ray image is formed when only indirect transmission photons reach the image receptor.
3. T F Coherent scattering does not contribute to radiographic fog in mammography because breast tissue is gently but firmly compressed during this imaging procedure.
4. T F During the process of Compton scattering, an x-ray photon interacts with an inner-shell electron of an atom of the irradiated object.
5. T F A photoelectron usually is absorbed within a few micrometers of the medium through which it travels, thereby increasing patient dose and contributing to biologic damage in tissue.
6. T F Absorption properties of different body structures must be identical to make diagnostically useful images possible.
7. T F The intensity of radiation scatter in various directions is a major factor in the planning of protection for medical imaging personnel during a radiologic examination.
8. T F Pair production is also known as *Rayleigh scattering*.
9. T F In the radiographic kilovoltage range, compact bone with a high calcium content by weight undergoes much more photoelectric absorption than an equal mass of soft tissue and air.
10. T F The use of positive contrast media leads to a decrease in absorbed dose in the body structures that contain them.
11. T F Compton scattering results in all-directional scatter.
12. T F A Compton-scattered electron is also known as an *Auger electron*.
13. T F Rayleigh and Thompson types of scattering play essentially no role in radiography.
14. T F For each radiographic procedure, an optimal kVp and mAs combination exists that minimizes the dose to the patient and produces an acceptable radiographic image.
15. T F A photoelectron may interact with other atoms, but it cannot cause excitation or ionization of those atoms.
16. T F *Attenuation* is any process that increases the intensity of the primary photon beam directed toward a destination.
17. T F During the process of photoelectric absorption, the atom also emits primary radiation when the outer-shell electron fills the inner-shell vacancy.
18. T F The minimum energy required to produce an electron-positron pair is 0.022 megaelectron volts (MeV).
19. T F The target in the x-ray tube is also known as the *cathode*.
20. T F If an electron is drawn across an electrical potential difference of 1 volt (V), it has acquired an energy of 1 eV.
21. T F The term *exit photons* is synonymous with the term *image formation photons*.
22. T F The byproducts of photoelectric absorption include photoelectrons and characteristic x-ray photons.
23. T F The effective atomic number (Z_{eff}) of air is 13.8.
24. T F Biologic damage in the patient may result from the absorption of x-ray energy.
25. T F kVp selection usually is based on the type of procedure and body part to be radiographed.

Exercise 5: Fill in the Blank
Using the following Word Bank, fill in the blanks with the word or words that best complete the statements.

absorption (term may be used more than once)	electrical voltage	kinetic
antimatter	electrons (term may be used more than once)	kVp
Auger		man-made
backward		one-third
coherent (classical, elastic, or unmodified) (term may be used more than once)	energy (term may be used more than once)	photoelectric (term may be used more than once)
	forward	
	image	
Compton (term may be used more than once)	increase	photons
	increases (term may be used more than once)	positively
darker		Rayleigh
decreases		recoil
degrade	intensity	Thompson

1. X-rays are carriers of _____, electromagnetic energy.

2. As _____ interact with the atoms of the target, x-ray _____ emerge from the target with a broad range of energies and leave the x-ray tube through a glass window.

3. The energy of the electrons inside the x-ray tube is expressed in terms of the _____ _____ applied across the tube.

4. In clinical situations, scattered photons reach the image receptor and _____ image quality.

5. In a diagnostic x-ray beam, the ultimate destination of photons is the _____ receptor.

6. In the process of _____ scattering, because the wavelengths of both incident and scattered waves are the same, no net energy has been absorbed by the atom.

7. Compton scatter may be directed _____ as small-angle scatter, _____ as backscatter, and to the side as sidescatter.

8. _____ scattering and _____ absorption in tissue are equally probable at about 35 keV.

9. When an inner-shell electron is removed from an atom in a photoelectric interaction, causing an inner-shell vacancy, the energy liberated when this vacancy is filled can, instead of emerging from the atom as fluorescent radiation, be transferred to another electron of the atom, thereby ejecting the electron. Such an emitted electron is called an _____ electron.

10. Biologic damage may result from the _____ of x-ray energy.

11. A diagnostic x-ray beam is produced when a stream of high-speed _____ bombard a _____-charged target in a highly evacuated glass tube.

12. Although all photons in a diagnostic x-ray beam do not have the same _____, the most energetic photons in the beam can have no more _____ than the electrons that bombard the target.

13. For a typical diagnostic x-ray unit, the energy of the average photon in the x-ray beam is about _____ _____ the energy of the most energetic photon.

14. The _____ of radiation scatter in various directions is a major factor in the planning of protection for medical imaging personnel during a radiologic examination.

15. _____ and _____ scattering play essentially no role in radiography.

16. The less a given structure attenuates radiation, the _____ its radiographic image will be, and vice versa.

17. Use of a positive contrast medium leads to an _____ in absorbed dose in the body structures that contain the medium.

18. A positron is classified as a form of _____.

19. The _____ effect is the basis of radiographic imaging, whereas the _____ effect is its bane.

20. _____ scattering is most likely to occur at below 10 keV.

21. When _____ is increased, the patient receives a lower radiation dose, but image quality may be compromised.

22. Within the energy range of diagnostic radiology that includes mammography (23 to 150 kVp), when kVp is decreased, the number of photoelectric interactions _____ and the number of Compton interactions _____; however, the patient absorbs more energy, and therefore the patient dose _____.

23. Variations in the x-ray _____ properties of various body structures make radiographic imaging of human anatomy possible.

24. A Compton-scattered electron is also known as a secondary, or _____, electron.

25. An incoming x-ray photon has _____ energy.

Exercise 6: Labeling
Label the following illustrations.

A. Primary, exit, and attenuated photons.

B. Process of Compton scattering.

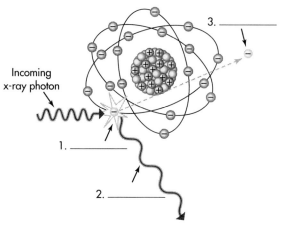

Primary − Exit = Attenuation

Chapter 2 Interaction of X-Radiation with Matter

C. Process of photoelectric absorption.

Exercise 7: Short Answer
Answer the following questions by providing a short answer.

1. Name five types of interaction that can occur between x-radiation and matter.

   _____

   _____

2. How is a radiographer actually responsible for a dose the patient receives during an x-ray procedure?

   _____

   _____

3. What is responsible for producing diagnostically useful images in which different anatomic structures can be perceived and distinguished?

4. How can the radiographer reduce the amount of radiographic fog produced by small-angle scatter?

5. How is the energy of the electrons inside a diagnostic x-ray tube expressed?

6. What is the minimum energy required to produce an electron-positron pair?

7. Of what do positive contrast media consist?

8. Name three unstable nuclei used in positron emission tomography (PET) scanning.

9. What type of energy does a photoelectron have?

10. What can happen to the radiographic image from scattered radiation?

11. List the two methods most commonly used to limit the effects of indirectly transmitted x-ray photons.

12. During the process of coherent scattering, why is no net energy absorbed by the atom with which the incident x-ray photon interacts?

13. What is mass density? How is it measured?

14. What is radiographic contrast?

15. In what radiation modality is annihilation radiation used?

Exercise 8: General Discussion or Opinion Questions

The following questions are intended to allow students to express their knowledge and understanding of the subject matter or to present a personal opinion. The questions may be used to stimulate class discussion. Because answers to these questions may vary, determination of an answer's acceptability is left to the discretion of the course instructor.

1. Discuss the importance of photoelectric absorption in radiography, and explain the impact of this x-ray interaction on the patient dose.

2. How can a radiographer limit the production of scattered radiation in a radiography room?

3. Discuss the use of positive contrast media in radiography. How does the use of such media affect patient dose?

4. Discuss the probability of photon interaction with matter.

5. How can radiographers select technical exposure factors for routine x-ray procedures to minimize the radiation dose to the patient and produce an optimal-quality image?

POST-TEST

The student should take this test after reading Chapter 2, finishing all accompanying textbook and workbook exercises, and completing any additional activities required by the course instructor. The student should complete the post-test with a score of 90% or higher before advancing to the next chapter. (Each of the following 20 questions or blanks is worth 5 points.) Score = _____%

1. Use of a barium- or iodine-based contrast medium significantly enhances the occurrence of _____ absorption in biologic tissue, resulting in an increase in the radiation dose to the patient.

2. Define the term *attenuation*.

3. For each radiographic procedure, an optimal kVp and mAs combination exists that _____ the dose to the patient and produces an optimal-quality image.

4. In fluoroscopy, Compton-scattered photons can expose imaging _____ who are present in the room.

5. During the process of Compton scattering, the energy of the incident x-ray photon is _____ absorbed.

6. What controls the quality, or penetrating power, of an x-ray beam?
   _____

7. The interaction of x-ray photons with any atoms of biologic matter are _____ in nature; therefore the effects of such interactions cannot be predicted with certainty.

8. Pair production and _____ do not occur within the range of diagnostic radiology.

9. Which interaction of x-radiation with matter is most responsible for the contrast between bone and soft tissue that is seen on an optimal-quality image?
   _____

10. Scattered radiation can result in:
    1. A higher-quality diagnostic image
    2. Exposure to personnel who are present in a fluoroscopic room during a procedure
    3. Radiographic fog
    A. 1 and 2 only
    B. 1 and 3 only
    C. 2 and 3 only
    D. 1, 2, and 3

11. A positron is considered:
    A. A form of antimatter
    B. A modified proton
    C. A form of small-angle scatter
    D. A byproduct of the photoelectric interaction

12. The symbol Z_{eff} indicates:
    A. Atomic number
    B. Effective atomic number
    C. Mass number
    D. The number of vacancies in an atomic shell

13. Which of the following x-radiation interactions with matter is most likely to occur at below 10 keV?
    A. Coherent scattering
    B. Compton scattering
    C. Photoelectric absorption
    D. Pair production

14. Which of the following terms are synonymous?
    A. Classical scattering and photoelectric absorption
    B. Compton scattering and photodisintegration
    C. Photoelectric absorption and Compton scattering
    D. Characteristic radiation and fluorescent radiation

15. PET makes use of:
    A. Annihilation radiation
    B. Compton-scattered photons
    C. Photoelectrons
    D. Bremsstrahlung

16. What is the effective atomic number of compact bone?

17. What term is used for the energy absorbed by the patient per unit mass?

18. To ensure the quality of the radiographic image and the patient's safety, both the radiologist and the radiographer should choose the highest-energy x-ray beam that permits adequate radiographic _____ for computed radiography, digital radiography, or conventional radiography.

19. Compton scattering results in _____ scatter.

20. To what does the term *fluorescent yield* refer?

3 Radiation Quantities and Units

Chapter 3 covers the evolution of radiation quantities and units. It also highlights the efforts made by medical professionals, since the harmful effects of x-rays became clear, to find a way to reduce radiation exposure throughout the world by developing standards for measuring and limiting such exposure. Diagnostic imaging personnel must be familiar with these standardized radiation quantities and units so that they can measure patient and personnel exposure consistently and uniformly.

CHAPTER HIGHLIGHTS

- Radiation units can be expressed in the International System of Units (SI) or the traditional system.
- Coulombs per kilogram (C/kg) or roentgens (R) is used for exposure in air only.
- The gray (Gy) or rad is used for absorbed dose (D) measurement.
- Equivalent dose (EqD) and effective dose (EfD) are the quantities of choice for measuring biologic effects when all types of radiation must be considered.
- EqD specifies how much biologic damage from different types and doses of radiation will be equivalent if correct weighting factors are included.
- EfD describes the way the same effective amount of damage can be attained by giving different equivalent doses to different organs.
- Sievert (Sv) and rem are the units of equivalent dose and effective dose.
- Collective effective dose (ColEfD) is used when calculating group or population radiation exposure from low doses of different sources of ionizing radiation.
- Person-sievert is the unit used to calculate the radiation quantity *collective effective dose*.
- To calculate equivalent dose: $EqD = D \times W_R$.
- To calculate effective dose: $EfD = D \times W_R \times W_T$.

Exercise 1: Crossword Puzzle

Use the clues to complete the crossword puzzle.

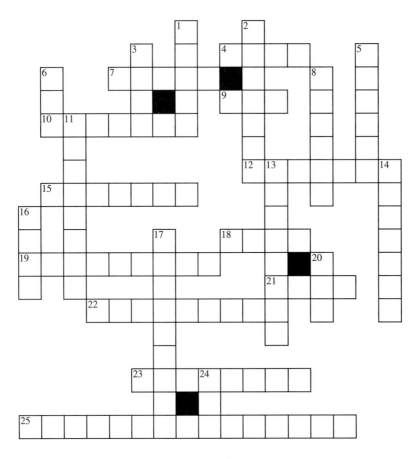

Down

1. First American radiation fatality
2. Biologic effects of ionizing radiation, or other agents, on generations yet unborn
3. Greek word meaning body
5. Weighting factor—that is, a conceptual measure for the relative risk associated with irradiation of different body tissues
6. Unit of energy and work
8. Fluoroscope inventor
11. Total electrical charge of one sign, either all pluses or all minuses, per unit mass that x-ray and gamma-ray photons with energies up to 3 million electron volts generate in dry, that is, nonhumid, air at standard temperature and pressure (760 mm Hg or 1 atmosphere at sea level and 220° C)
13. Traditional unit of the radiation quantity *exposure (X)*
14. Swedish physicist after whom the SI unit of equivalent dose was named
16. Type of somatic effect of ionizing radiation that appears months or years after exposure
17. Radiation dose to which occupationally exposed persons could be continuously subjected without any apparent harmful acute effects, such as erythema of the skin
20. Acronym for *radiation absorbed dose*
24. Acronym for *radiation equivalent man*

Across

4. Safe dose of ionizing radiation
7. The work done or energy expended when a force of 1 N acts on an object along a distance of 1 m
9. Concept that helps explain the need for a quality, or modifying, factor
10. Country in which x-rays were discovered
12. Pear-shaped, partial vacuum discharge tube
15. Basic unit of electrical charge
18. Part of human body imaged on the world's first x-ray picture on film
19. Dose of radiation below which an individual has a negligible chance of sustaining specific biologic damage
21. SI unit of D
22. Dose that provides a measure of the overall risk of exposure to ionizing radiation
23. Patient's skin surface where radiation dose received will be highest
25. Reddening of the skin of early radiologists and dentists caused by exposure to ionizing radiation

Exercise 2: Matching
Match the following terms with their definitions or associated phrases.

1. _____ aplastic anemia
2. _____ linear energy transfer (LET)
3. _____ SI
4. _____ leukemia
5. _____ rad
6. _____ somatic damage
7. _____ Gy
8. _____ rem
9. _____ R
10. _____ person-sievert
11. _____ W_R
12. _____ occupational exposure
13. _____ EfD
14. _____ Crookes tube
15. _____ gamma radiation
16. _____ skin erythema dose
17. _____ EqD
18. _____ *soma*
19. _____ Sv
20. _____ D
21. _____ Bragg–Gray theory
22. _____ barium platinocyanide
23. _____ exposure
24. _____ traditional units
25. _____ effective atomic number (Z_{eff})

A. Unit used from 1900 to 1930 to measure radiation exposure
B. The traditional unit for the radiation quantity, equivalent dose
C. Allows units to be used interchangeably among all branches of science throughout the world
D. Concept that helps explain the need for a quality, or modifying, factor
E. Unit that has been used traditionally to express D
F. SI unit of EqD
G. Blood disorder resulting in abnormal overproduction of white blood cells after exposure to ionizing radiation
H. The product of $D \times W_R \times W_T$
I. Relates the ionization produced in a small cavity within an irradiated medium or object to the energy absorbed in that medium as a result of its radiation exposure
J. Blood disorder resulting from bone marrow failure after exposure to ionizing radiation
K. Product of $D \times W_R$
L. Biologic damage to the body caused by exposure to ionizing radiation
M. SI unit for the radiation quantity ColEfD
N. Radiation exposure received by radiation workers in the course of exercising their professional responsibilities
O. SI unit used to express D
P. Greek term meaning body
Q. The amount of ionizing radiation that may strike an object such as the human body when in the vicinity of a radiation source
R. Special units associated with radiation protection and dosimetry, namely the roentgen and the rem
S. A dimensionless factor (a multiplier) that was chosen for radiation protection purposes to account for differences in biologic impact among various types of ionizing radiation
T. A pear-shaped, partial vacuum discharge tube
U. Fluorescent material that coated the paper used when x-rays were discovered
V. A composite, or weighted average, of the atomic numbers of the many different chemical elements that comprise a given biologic tissue
W. Short wavelength, higher energy electromagnetic waves emitted by the nuclei of radioactive substances
X. The amount of energy per unit mass absorbed by an irradiated object
Y. The photon (either x-ray or gamma ray) exposure that under standard conditions of pressure and temperature produces a total positive or negative ion charge of 2.58×10^{-4} C/kg of dry air

Exercise 3: Multiple Choice

Select the answer that *best* completes the following questions or statements.

1. Which of the following factors must be multiplied to determine the EfD from an x-radiation exposure of an organ or body part?
   A. EqD × W_R × D
   B. W_T × W_R × ColEfD
   C. D × W_R × W_T
   D. D × C/kg

2. Which of the following is the SI unit of radiation exposure?
   A. C/kg
   B. Gy
   C. R
   D. Sv

3. The expression 10^{-6} may be *symbolically* expressed as which of the following?
   A. π
   B. Ω
   C. Σ
   D. μ

4. In radiation protection systems no longer in use, a radiation dose to which occupationally exposed persons could be continuously subjected *without* any apparent harmful acute effects, such as erythema of the skin, was known as a(n):
   A. Effective dose
   B. Maximum permissible dose
   C. Tolerance dose
   D. Weighted dose

5. Short-term somatic effects of radiation include:
   1. Nausea and fatigue
   2. Blood and intestinal disorders
   3. Diffuse redness of the skin and shedding of its outer layer
   A. 1 and 2 only
   B. 1 and 3 only
   C. 2 and 3 only
   D. 1, 2, and 3

6. Which of the following terms describes the amount of energy per unit mass transferred from an x-ray beam to an object in its path such as the human body?
   A. SI
   B. Exposure
   C. Equivalent dose
   D. Absorbed dose

7. To determine D, the amount of energy absorbed by the irradiated object must be measured by:
   A. Calculating the EqD
   B. Calculating the entrance skin exposure of the object
   C. Determining the amount of energy deposited per kilogram of the irradiated object
   D. Determining the amount of ionization in a specified volume of dry air at atmospheric pressure

8. LET is expressed in units of:
   A. EfD
   B. EqD
   C. keV/μm
   D. Person-sievert

9. The EfD is based on which of the following?
   A. The energy deposited in biologic tissue by ionizing radiation
   B. The electrical charge produced in a kilogram of dry air by ionizing radiation
   C. The dose of ionizing radiation required to cause diffuse redness over an area of skin
   D. The number of electron-ion pairs in a specific volume of air

10. Which of the following is the radiation unit used for x-ray equipment calibration in which x-ray output is measured directly with an ionization chamber?
    A. Sv (rem)
    B. Gy (rad)
    C. rem (rom)
    D. C/kg (R)

11. Which of the following radiation quantities can be used to compare the average amount of radiation received by the entire body from a specific radiologic examination with the amount received from natural background radiation?
    A. D
    B. EfD
    C. EqD
    D. Exposure

12. Which of the following radiation quantities is used to describe population or group exposure to low doses of different sources of ionizing radiation?
    A. D
    B. EqD
    C. Exposure
    D. ColEfD

13. A W_R has been established for the following ionizing radiations: x-rays (W_R = 1); fast neutrons (W_R = 20); and alpha particles (W_R = 20). What is the *total* EqD (in rem) for a person who has received the following exposures: x-rays = 4 rad; fast neutrons = 6 rad; and alpha particles = 3 rad?
    A. 1.84
    B. 18.4
    C. 184
    D. 1840

14. A dimensionless factor, or multiplier, that places risks associated with biologic effects on a common scale is known as the:
    A. D
    B. Background time factor
    C. EqD
    D. W_R

15. Which of the following have similar numeric values?
    1. Quality factor (Q)
    2. W_R
    3. W_T
    A. 1 and 2 only
    B. 1 and 3 only
    C. 2 and 3 only
    D. 1, 2, and 3

16. If a patient undergoing x-ray therapy receives a total dose of 3000 rad, the dose may be recorded as _____ if the SI system is used.
    A. 6000 Gy
    B. 3000 centigray (cGy)
    C. 300 rad
    D. 30 R

17. Which of the following types of radiation has a W_R of 20?
    A. Alpha particles
    B. Gamma radiation
    C. Neutrons, energy <10 keV
    D. X-radiation

18. Ten sievert equal _____ rem.
    A. 10
    B. 100
    C. 1000
    D. 10,000

19. Which of the following is (are) equivalent to 1 rem?
    1. $1/100$ Sv
    2. 1 centisievert (cSv)
    3. 10 millisievert (mSv)
    A. 1 only
    B. 2 only
    C. 3 only
    D. 1, 2, and 3

20. Thomas A. Edison invented the:
    A. Cold cathode x-ray tube
    B. Hot cathode x-ray tube
    C. Fluoroscope
    D. Standard ionization chamber

21. Which of the following is or are *not* traditional units?
    A. C/kg
    B. Gy and Sv
    C. R, rad, rem
    D. A and B

22. The ampere is the SI unit of:
    A. Electrical charge
    B. Electrical current
    C. Electrical resistance
    D. X-ray ionization in air

23. One rad is equivalent to an energy transfer of:
    A. 500 erg per gram of irradiated object
    B. 300 erg per gram of irradiated object
    C. 200 erg per gram of irradiated object
    D. 100 erg per gram of irradiated object

24. X-rays, beta particles (high-speed electrons), and gamma rays have been given a numeric adjustment value of 1 because they produce:
    A. No biologic effect in body tissue for equal absorbed doses
    B. Varying degrees of biologic effect in body tissue for equal absorbed doses
    C. High-dose biologic effects in all body tissues for even the smallest dose
    D. Virtually the same biologic effect in body tissue for equal absorbed doses

25. In therapeutic radiology, which of the following units is replacing the rad for recording of the absorbed dose?
    A. cGy
    B. milligray (mGy)
    C. mSv
    D. Sv

Exercise 4: True or False

Circle *T* if the statement is true; circle *F* if the statement is false.

1. T F Wilhelm Conrad Roentgen discovered x-rays on November 8, 1895, at the University of Wurzburg in Bavaria, Germany.

2. T F When x-rays were discovered, a charge was being passed through a pear-shaped, partial vacuum discharge tube. Light was seen emanating from a piece of paper coated with calcium tungstate that lay on a bench several feet away.

3. T F Cancer deaths among physicians attributed to x-ray exposure were reported as early as 1910.

4. T F The British X-ray and Radium Protection Committee was formed in 1921 to investigate methods for reducing radiation exposure because medical professionals were alarmed by the increasing number of radiation injuries reported.

5. T F By the 1950s EfD had replaced the tolerance dose for radiation protection purposes.

6. T F In 1991 tissue weighting factors were revised by the NCRP based on data from more recent epidemiologic studies of the Chernobyl survivors.

7. T F   Fluoroscopic entrance exposure rates are measured in roentgens per minute (R/min), and essentially all radiation survey instruments provide readings in traditional units.

8. T F   The SI unit of absorbed dose, the gray, was named after the English radiobiologist Dorian Gray.

9. T F   The ampere is the SI unit of electrical current.

10. T F   Sv and R are the units used in the calculation of the radiation quantities EqD and EfD.

11. T F   C/kg or R is used for measurement of the D.

12. T F   In radiation therapy, the cGy is replacing the rad for recording of the D.

13. T F   Each type and energy of radiation has a specific W_R.

14. T F   As the intensity of x-ray exposure of an air volume increases, the number of electron-ion pairs produced decreases.

15. T F   Absorbed energy is responsible for any biologic damage caused by exposure of tissues to radiation.

16. T F   Skin erythema dose was an accurate means of measuring radiation exposure because the same amount of radiation produced erythema in all patients.

17. T F   In 1991 the ICRP revised tissue weighting factors based on data from more recent epidemiologic studies of atomic bomb survivors.

18. T F   The EfD is based on the energy deposited in biologic tissue by ionizing radiation.

19. T F   The lower the atomic number of a material, the more x-ray energy it absorbs.

20. T F   Radiation weighting factors are selected by national and international scientific advisory bodies (NCRP, ICRP) and are based on quality factors and linear energy transfer.

21. T F   The EqD for measuring biologic effects may be determined and expressed in C/kg (SI system) or in R (traditional system).

22. T F   The concept of tolerance dose was originally developed to protect occupationally exposed persons from acute affects of radiation exposure.

23. T F   Sv or rem is used for the D measurement.

24. T F   The EfD can be expressed in Sv or mSv.

25. T F   By the 1970s dosimetry and risk analysis had become quite sophisticated.

Exercise 5: Fill in the Blank

Using the following Word Bank, fill in the blanks with the word or words that best complete the statements.

0.1	ionization (charge)	Rolf Maxmilian Sievert
0.2	Louis Harold Gray	roentgen (term may be used more than once)
absorbed dose	measure	
biologic effect	nonhazardous	safety
cancerous	organs	SI
coulomb	organ systems	sieverts
different	pressure	temperature
entire	quantities	units
erythema	radiation equivalent man	Wilhelm Conrad Roentgen
exposure	rem	workable
humidity	risk	

1. In late November 1895, _____ _____ took the world's first x-ray picture on film, which clearly showed the bones of his wife's hand.

2. Many of the skin lesions on the hands and fingers of early radiologists and dentists eventually became _____ as a consequence of continued exposure to ionizing radiation.

3. Because the amount of radiation required to produce the _____ reaction varied from one person to another, it was a crude and inaccurate way to measure radiation exposure.

4. In 1937 the roentgen was accepted internationally as the unit of measurement for _____ to x-radiation and gamma radiation.

5. By the 1970s recognition was growing that the health consequences for the human body as a whole organism depended on which _____ and _____ _____ had been irradiated.

6. _____ _____ is the deposition of energy per unit mass by ionizing radiation in the patient's body tissue.

7. A _____ represents the amount of electrical charge flowing past a point in a circuit in 1 second when an electrical current of 1 ampere is used.

8. X-rays, beta particles (high-speed electrons), and gamma rays produce virtually the same _____ _____ in body tissue for equal absorbed doses.

9. The EqD for measuring biologic effects may be determined and expressed in _____ or in _____.

10. The W_T accounts for the _____ to the _____ organism brought on by irradiation of individual tissues and organs.

11. Rem is an acronym for _____ _____ _____.

12. Trade or government desk work is considered a(n) _____ occupation.

13. By the 1970s, radiation units were developed that included factors that accounted for the varied biologic effects of _____ types of radiation.

14. To be able to measure patient and personnel exposure in a consistent and uniform manner, diagnostic imaging personnel should be familiar with the radiation _____ and _____.

15. In 1921 the British X-ray and Radium Protection Committee was formed to investigate methods for reducing radiation exposure. The members of the committee were unable to fulfill their responsibility because they could not agree on a _____ unit of radiation exposure.

16. The _____ was the principal guideline for occupational radiation exposure during the 1930s.

17. In 1934 the U.S. Advisory Committee on X-Ray and Radium Protection recommended a tolerance dose equal to _____ R/day. In 1936 the committee reduced this dose to _____ R/day.

18. In 1937 the _____ became internationally accepted as the unit of measurement for exposure to x-radiation and gamma radiation; in 1962 this unit was redefined to improve accuracy and acceptability.

19. Neither tolerance dose nor threshold dose is currently being used for the purposes of radiation _____.

20. The International Commission on Radiation Units and Measurements (ICRU) adopted _____ units for use with ionizing radiation in 1980 and urged full implementation of these units as soon as possible.

21. _____ was instrumental in developing the most important theory of radiation dosimetry.

22. _____ is best known for his method for determining the exposure rates at various points near linear radium sources (tubes).

23. Each radiation quantity has a particular unit of _____.

24. For precise measurement of radiation exposure in radiography, the total amount of _____ an x-ray beam produces in a known mass of air must be obtained.

25. A standard or free air ionization chamber contains a known amount of air with precisely measured _____, _____, and _____.

Exercise 6: Labeling

Label the following illustration and tables.

A. Standard or free air ionization chamber.

B. Radiation weighting factors for different types and energies of ionizing radiation.

Radiation Type and Energy Range	Radiation Weighting Factor (W_R)
X-ray and gamma ray photons, electrons (every energy)	1. _____
Neutrons, energy < 10 keV	2. _____
10-100 keV	3. _____
>100 keV to 2 MeV	4. _____
>2-20 MeV	5. _____
>20 MeV	6. _____
Protons	7. _____
Alpha particles	8. _____

Data adapted from International Commission on Radiological Protection (ICRP): *Recommendations,* ICRP Publication No. 60, New York, 1991, Pergamon Press.

C. Summary of radiation quantities and units.

Type of Radiation	Quantity	SI Unit	Traditional Unit	Measuring Medium	Radiation Effect Measured
X-radiation or gamma	1. _____	Coulomb per kilogram (C/kg)	Roentgen (R)	Air	Ionization of air radiation
All ionizing radiations	2. _____	Gray (Gy)	Rad	Any object	Amount of energy per unit mass absorbed by object
All ionizing radiations	3. _____	Sievert (Sv)	Rem	Body tissue	Biologic effects
All ionizing radiations	4. _____	Sievert (Sv)	Rem	Body tissue	Biologic effects

Exercise 7: Short Answer

Answer the following questions by providing a short answer.

1. Why did Thomas A. Edison discontinue his x-ray research?

2. What unit was used for measuring radiation exposure from 1900 to 1930?

3. What is the difference between the short-term and the long-term somatic effects of ionizing radiation?

4. What is a tolerance dose?

5. What unit replaced the tolerance dose for radiation protection purposes in the 1950s?

6. In the late 1970s, dose limits were calculated and established to ensure what?

7. What is the Bragg-Gray theory, and what significance does it have?

8. When the human body is exposed to ionizing radiation, for what is absorbed energy responsible?

9. For a precise measurement of radiation exposure in radiography, what must be obtained?

10. Who is responsible for selecting radiation weighting factors, and on what are these factors based?

11. If D is stated in rad, how is the equivalent in Gy determined?

12. If D is stated in Gy, how is the equivalent in rad determined?

13. What SI and traditional units of measure are used for x-ray equipment calibration? Why are these units used?

14. If radiation exposure is given in R, how can that value be converted to C/kg?

15. If radiation exposure is given in C/kg, how can that value be converted to R?

Exercise 8: General Discussion or Opinion Questions

The following questions are intended to allow students to express their knowledge and understanding of the subject matter or to present a personal opinion. The questions may be used to stimulate class discussion. Because answers to these questions may vary, determination of an answer's acceptability is left to the discretion of the course instructor.

1. How were x-rays discovered?

2. How did occupational radiation exposure affect the pioneers of the radiation industry?

3. What problems did medical professionals encounter as they investigated methods for reducing radiation exposure in the early 1900s?

4. What changes in radiation protection criteria led to the use of EfD and EqD for radiation protection purposes?

5. Explain the equivalence of damage caused by radiation from different sources of ionizing radiation.

6. Explain the significance and use of a W_R.

7. Explain the significance and use of a W_T.

8. Summarize the radiation quantities and units currently in use.

9. Discuss the concept of LET and its significance.

10. Discuss the use of SI units in the field of radiology.

Exercise 9: Calculation Problems

Using the information presented below, set up and solve the following problems.

A. The SI unit of the radiation quantity D is the Gy; the traditional unit is the rad. Gy and rad units are easily converted to allow comparison of D values. If D is stated in rad, the equivalent in Gy can be determined by dividing the rad value by 100. If D is stated in Gy, rad can be determined by multiplying the Gy value by 100.

1. Convert 8000 rad to Gy.

2. Convert 8 rad to Gy.

3. Convert 450 rad to Gy.

4. Convert 4.5 rad to Gy.

5. Convert 375 rad to Gy.

6. Convert 7 Gy to rad.

7. Convert 25 Gy to rad.

8. Convert 0.4 Gy to rad.

9. Convert 0.087 Gy to rad.

10. Convert 0.96 Gy to rad.

B. EqD is used for radiation protection purposes when a person receives exposure from various types of ionizing radiation. The EqD for measuring biologic effects can be determined and expressed in Sv (SI units) or rem (traditional units). The EqD is obtained by multiplying D by W_R.

1. A W_R has been established for each of the following ionizing radiations: x-radiation ($W_R = 1$); fast neutrons ($W_R = 20$); and alpha particles ($W_R = 20$). What is the total EqD in Sv for a person who has received the following exposures: x-radiation = 0.6 Gy; fast neutrons = 0.25 Gy; and alpha particles = 0.4 Gy?

2. A W_R has been established for each of the following ionizing radiations: x-radiation ($W_R = 1$); fast neutrons ($W_R = 20$); gamma rays ($W_R = 1$); protons ($W_R = 2$); and alpha particles ($W_R = 20$). What is the total EqD in Sv for a person who has received the following exposures: x-radiation = 0.3 Gy; fast neutrons = 0.28 Gy; gamma rays = 0.8 Gy; protons = 0.9 Gy; and alpha particles = 0.4 Gy?

3. A W_R has been established for each of the following ionizing radiations: x-radiation ($W_R = 1$); fast neutrons ($W_R = 20$); and alpha particles ($W_R = 20$). What is the total EqD in rem for a person who has received the following exposures: x-radiation = 7 rad; fast neutrons = 2 rad; and alpha particles = 5 rad?

4. A W_R has been established for each of the following ionizing radiations: x-radiation ($W_R = 1$); fast neutrons ($W_R = 20$); gamma rays ($W_R = 1$); protons ($W_R = 2$); and alpha particles ($W_R = 20$). What is the total EqD in rem for a person who has received the following exposures: x-radiation = 3 rad; fast neutrons = 0.35 rad; gamma rays = 6 rad; protons = 2.5 rad; and alpha particles = 8 rad?

5. A W_R has been established for each of the following ionizing radiations: x-radiation ($W_R = 1$); fast neutrons, energy = 10 keV ($W_R = 5$); gamma rays ($W_R = 1$); protons ($W_R = 2$); and alpha particles ($W_R = 20$). What is the total EqD in Sv for a person who has received the following exposures: x-radiation = 0.6 Gy; fast neutrons, energy = 10 keV = 0.2 Gy; gamma rays = 4 Gy; protons = 0.8 Gy; and alpha particles = 6 Gy?

C. The EfD is a quantity used for radiation protection purposes to provide a measure of the overall risk of exposure to ionizing radiation. It incorporates both the effect of the type of radiation used (e.g., x-radiation, gamma, neutron) and the variability in radiosensitivity of the organ or body part irradiated through the use of appropriate weighting factors. These factors determine the overall harm to these biologic components for risk of developing a radiation-induced cancer or, in the case of the reproductive organs, genetic damage. The formula for determining the EfD is as follows: EfD = $D \times W_R \times W_T$. The EfD may be expressed in Sv (SI units) or rem (traditional units).

1. The W_R for alpha particles is 20, and the W_T for the breast is 0.05. If the breast receives a D of 0.5 Gy from exposure to alpha particles, what is the EfD in Sv?

2. The W_R for x-radiation is 1, and the W_T for the gonads is 0.2. If the gonads receive a D of 0.4 Gy from exposure to x-radiation, what is the EfD in Sv?

3. The W_R for fast neutrons is 20, and the W_T for the stomach is 0.12. If the stomach receives a D of 6 rad from exposure to fast neutrons, what is the EfD in rem?

4. The W_R for gamma rays is 1, and the W_T for the esophagus is 0.05. If the esophagus receives a D of 25 rad from exposure to gamma rays, what is the EfD in rem?

5. The W_R for x-radiation is 1, and the W_T for red bone marrow is 0.12. If the red bone marrow receives a D of 0.9 Gy from exposure to x-radiation, what is the EfD in Sv?

D. In addition to EqD and EfD, another dosimetric quantity, the ColEfD, has been derived and implemented for use in radiation protection to describe internal and external dose measurements. Collective effective dose is used to describe radiation exposure of a population or group to low doses of different sources of ionizing radiation. It is the product of the average EfD for an individual belonging to the exposed population or group and the number of persons exposed. Therefore ColEfD is found by multiplying the average EfD for an individual belonging to the exposed population or group by the number of individuals exposed. The radiation unit for the ColEfD is the person-sievert (the man-rem formerly was used and is obtained by multiplying the person-sievert by 100).

1. If 400 people receive an average EfD of 0.2 Sv (20 rem), what is the ColEfD in person-sievert (and man-rem)?

2. If 300 people receive an average EfD of 0.17 Sv (17 rem), what is the ColEfD in person-sievert (and man-rem)?

3. If 250 people receive an average EfD of 0.24 Sv (24 rem), what is the ColEfD in person-sievert (and man-rem)?

4. If 1000 people receive an average EfD of 0.10 Sv (10 rem), what is the ColEfD in person-sievert (and man-rem)?

5. If 100 people receive an average EfD of 0.30 Sv (30 rem), what is the ColEfD in person-sievert (and man-rem)?

POST-TEST

The student should take this test after reading Chapter 3, finishing all accompanying textbook and workbook exercises, and completing any additional activities required by the course instructor. The student should complete the post-test with a score of 90% or higher before advancing to the next chapter. (Each of the following 20 questions or blanks is worth 5 points.) Score = _____ %

1. If 400 people receive an average EfD of 0.2 Sv (20 rem), what is the ColEfD in person-sievert (and man-rem)?

2. Which radiation quantity can be used to compare the average amount of radiation received by the entire body from a specific radiologic examination with the amount received from natural background radiation?

3. What concept helps explain the need for a radiation quality or modifying factor?

4. In what SI unit and in what traditional unit is the radiation quantity *exposure* (X) expressed?

5. _____ is a blood disorder resulting in abnormal overproduction of white blood cells after exposure to ionizing radiation.

6. Who is credited with discovering x-rays on November 8, 1895?

7. A W_R has been established for each of the following ionizing radiations: x-radiation ($W_R = 1$); fast neutrons ($W_R = 20$); and alpha particles ($W_R = 20$). What is the total EqD in Sv for a person who has received the following exposures: x-radiation = 5 Gy; fast neutrons = 0.3 Gy; and alpha particles = 0.7 Gy?

8. The W_R for x-radiation is 1, and the W_T for the lungs is 0.12. If the lungs receive a D of 5 Gy from exposure to x-radiation, what is the EfD in Sv?

9. Eight sievert equals _____ rem.

10. How is the EqD calculated?

11. The amount of energy per unit mass absorbed by the irradiated object is the definition of
    A. D
    B. EfD
    C. EqD
    D. X

12. The effective atomic number of bone is
    A. 7.4
    B. 7.6
    C. 13.8
    D. 20

13. _____ _____ was used as the first measure of exposure for ionizing radiation.

14. What is the basic unit of electrical charge?
    _____

15. Which of the following are short-term somatic effects of ionizing radiation?
    1. Diffuse redness of the skin
    2. Blood and intestinal disorders
    3. Nausea and vomiting
    A. 1 and 2 only
    B. 1 and 3 only
    C. 2 and 3 only
    D. 1, 2, and 3

16. One rem equals _____ mSv.

17. In radiation therapy, what SI subunit is replacing the rad for the recording of D?
    _____

18. Many of the skin lesions on the hands and fingers of early radiologists and dentists eventually became _____ as a consequence of continued exposure to ionizing radiation.

19. Define the term *occupational exposure*.
    _____
    _____

20. On what is the EfD based?
    _____
    _____

4 Radiation Monitoring

Chapter 4 covers radiation monitoring, both personnel monitoring and area monitoring. Personnel exposure must be monitored to ensure that occupational radiation exposure levels are kept well below the annual effective dose (EfD) limit. Specific gas-filled radiation detectors that serve as field instruments detect the presence of radiation and, when properly calibrated, give a reasonably accurate measurement of the exposure. Radiographers and other occupationally exposed persons must be aware of the various personnel and area radiation exposure monitoring devices and their functions.

CHAPTER HIGHLIGHTS

- Personnel monitoring ensures that occupational radiation exposure levels are kept well below the annual effective dose limit.
  - Personnel monitoring is required whenever radiation workers are likely to risk receiving 10% or more of the annual occupational effective dose limit of 50 mSv (5 rem) in any one year as a consequence of their work-related activities.
  - To keep radiation exposure as low as reasonably achievable (ALARA), most health care facilities issue dosimeter devices when personnel might receive about 1% of the annual occupational effective dose limit in any month, or approximately 0.5 mSv (50 mrem).
  - The working habits and conditions of diagnostic imaging personnel can be assessed over a designated period of time through the use of the personnel dosimeter.
  - A radiation worker should wear a personnel monitoring device at collar level during routine computed radiography, digital radiography, or conventional radiographic procedures to approximate the maximum radiation dose to the thyroid, head, and neck.
  - During high-level radiation procedures, imaging professionals should wear a protective lead apron, with the dosimeter worn outside of the garment at collar level, to provide a reading of the approximate equivalent dose to the thyroid and eyes.
  - During special computed radiography, digital radiography, or conventional radiographic procedures, two separate personnel dosimeters may be worn—a primary dosimeter worn outside the apron at collar level and a second dosimeter worn beneath the apron at waist level to monitor the approximate equivalent dose to the lower trunk.
  - Pregnant radiation workers should wear a second dosimeter to monitor the abdomen during gestation to provide an estimate of the equivalent dose to the embryo-fetus.
  - TLD ring badges are worn under certain conditions to monitor and determine equivalent dose to the hands when they are near the primary beam.
  - Health care facilities must maintain a record of exposure recorded by personnel dosimeters as part of each radiation worker's employment record.
  - In general, personnel dosimeters must be portable, durable, and cost-efficient.
  - Four types of personnel monitoring devices are available: film badges, OSL dosimeters, pocket ionization chambers, and TLDs.
  - To meet state and federal regulations, results from personnel monitoring programs must be recorded accurately and maintained by each health care facility.
  - The radiation safety officer (RSO) in a health care facility receives and reviews personnel monitoring reports to assess compliance with ALARA guidelines.
  - Monitoring reports list the deep, eye, and shallow occupational exposure of each person wearing a monitoring device in the facility, as measured by the exposed monitors.
- Area monitoring can be accomplished through the use of radiation survey instruments.
  - A simple detection system (e.g., just a GM tube with no quantitative readout device) will indicate only the presence or absence of radiation, whereas a dosimeter system (i.e., a detector plus a readout device) can quantitatively indicate both cumulative radiation intensity and radiation intensity rates.
  - Radiation survey instruments for area monitoring must be durable and easy to carry, be able to detect all common types of ionizing radiation, and not be affected by the energy of the radiation or the direction of the incident radiation.
  - Three types of gas-filled radiation survey instruments include the ionization chamber–type survey meter (cutie pie), the proportional counter, and the Geiger-Müller (GM) detector.
  - Radiographic and fluoroscopic units can be calibrated with ionization chambers. When used for this purpose, the ionization chamber is connected to an electrometer that can measure tiny electrical currents with high precision and accuracy.

Exercise 1: Crossword Puzzle

Use the clues to complete the crossword puzzle.

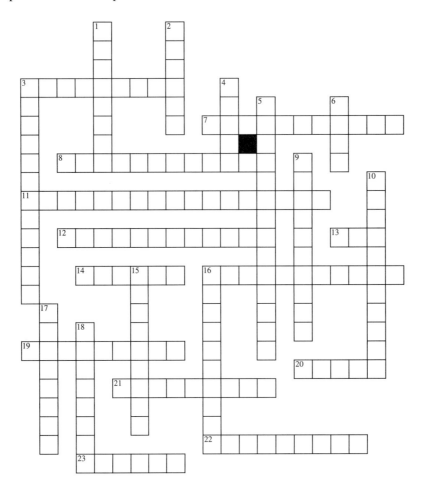

Down

1. A record of this should become part of the employment record of all radiation workers.
2. During routine computed radiography, digital radiography, or conventional radiographic procedures, when a protective apron is not being used, the primary personnel dosimeter should be attached to the clothing on the front of the body at this level to approximate the location of maximal radiation dose to the thyroid and the head and neck.
3. Type of counters not used in diagnostic imaging.
4. What the meter in an ionization chamber–type survey meter does without adequate warm-up time.
5. A graph or curve that represents the response of an image receptor to some probe.
6. Range of radiation exposure measured by a cutie pie within a few seconds.
9. Something that is recommended for any person occupationally exposed regularly to ionizing radiation.
10. A type of diagnostic imaging procedure where higher occupational exposure can be received.
15. Type of legal record of personnel exposure provided by a monitoring company reporting film badge or OSL dosimeter exposure.
16. Columns on a radiation dosimetry report that provide a continuous audit of actual absorbed radiation equivalent dose.
17. An outside influence that should not affect the performance of a radiation monitor worn by an occupationally exposed person.
18. What exposure monitoring of personnel is whenever radiation workers are likely to risk receiving 10% or more of the annual occupational effective dose limit of 50 mSv (5 rem) in any one year as a consequence of their work-related activities.

Across

3. Type of dosimeter used to monitor occupational radiation exposure for individuals.
7. A desirable characteristic for a dosimeter that is used to monitor a person's occupational radiation exposure.
8. A device that measures electrical charge.
11. The readout process destroys the stored information in this personnel dosimeter.
12. Word represented by the letter *L* in *OSL*.
13. Number of months an OSL dosimeter is commonly worn.
14. A metal of which a filter in a film badge is made.
16. What G-M detector tubes tend to lose over time.
19. Type of readout obtained when a pocket ionization chamber is used.
20. If a radiographer wearing a film badge stands too close to a patient during an exposure, this is how the image of the filters in the film badge will appear after the film has been developed.
21. Pregnant diagnostic imaging personnel should be issued a second monitoring device to record the radiation dose to the abdomen during this period of time.
22. Type of dosimeter that includes the TLD ring badge.
23. What radiation interacting with the film in a badge causes the film to do once it has been developed.

Exercise 2: Matching

Match the following terms with their definitions or associated phrases.

1. _____ personnel dosimeter
2. _____ personnel monitoring report
3. _____ radiation survey instruments
4. _____ OSL
5. _____ second personnel monitoring device
6. _____ Geiger-Müller detector
7. _____ control badge
8. _____ proportional counter
9. _____ optical density
10. _____ ionization chamber connected to an electrometer
11. _____ glow curve
12. _____ check source
13. _____ aluminum oxide (Al_2O_3) detector
14. _____ radiation-dosimetry film
15. _____ exposure monitoring of personnel
16. _____ densitometer

A. The intensity of light transmitted through a given area of the dosimetry film
B. Serves as a basis for comparison with the remaining badges after they have been returned to the monitoring company for processing
C. Device for monitoring occupational exposure that contains an Al_2O_3 detector
D. Resembles an ordinary fountain pen but contains a thimble ionization chamber that measures radiation exposure
E. Cutie pie
F. Contains LiF powder or chips, which function as a sensing material
G. Measures the amount of ionizing radiation to which a TLD badge has been exposed
H. Worn by a pregnant radiographer to monitor the equivalent dose to the embryo-fetus
I. Used to calibrate radiographic and fluoroscopic units
J. Economical type of personnel monitoring device that records whole-body radiation exposure accumulated at a low rate over a long period
K. Provides an indication of the working habits and working conditions of diagnostic imaging personnel
L. Specific gas-filled radiation detectors that detect the presence of radiation and, when properly calibrated, give a reasonably accurate measurement of the exposure
M. Lists the deep, eye, and shallow occupational exposures of each person in a health care facility as measured by the exposed monitor
N. Device with an audible system that alerts the operator to the presence of ionizing radiation
O. Generally used in laboratories to detect alpha and beta radiation and small amounts of other types of low-level radioactive contamination
P. Radiographic film in a film badge that is sensitive to doses ranging from as low as 0.1 mSv (10 mrem) to as high as 5000 mSv (500 rem)

17. _____ pocket dosimeter
18. _____ TLD analyzer
19. _____ ionization chamber–type survey meter
20. _____ TLD
21. _____ film badge
22. _____ lithium fluoride (LiF)
23. _____ ALARA policy
24. _____ fluoroscopy and special procedures
25. _____ TLD ring badge

Q. An instrument that can be used to determine the amount of radiation to which a film badge dosimeter has been exposed
R. Sensing material found in OSL dosimeters
S. Sensing material found in TLDs
T. Extremity monitor worn by an imaging professional as a second monitor when performing radiographic procedures that require the hands to be near the primary x-ray beam
U. Required whenever radiation workers are likely to risk receiving 10% or more of the annual EfD limit of 50 mSv (5 rem) in any one year as a consequence of their work-related activities
V. Areas of diagnostic radiology that produce the highest occupational radiation exposure for diagnostic imaging personnel
W. A weak, long-lived radioisotope located on the external surface of a GM detector that is used to verify the daily consistency of the unit
X. Keeping radiation exposure to personnel as low as reasonably achievable
Y. A graphical plot that demonstrates the relationship of light output, or emitted thermoluminescence intensity, to temperature variation

Exercise 3: Multiple Choice

Select the answer that best completes the following questions or statements.

1. In keeping with the ALARA concept, *most* health care facilities issue personnel dosimetry devices when personnel might receive about _____ of the annual occupational EfD limit in any 1 month, or approximately 0.5 mSv (50 mrem).
   A. 25%
   B. 10%
   C. 5%
   D. 1%

2. Which of the following will a simple detection system of a radiation survey instrument (e.g., just a GM tube with no quantitative readout device) do?
   A. It indicates cumulative radiation intensity and radiation intensity rates.
   B. It indicates only the presence or absence of radiation.
   C. It counts uncharged particles.
   D. A and C

3. Diagnostic imaging personnel should wear a personnel dosimeter during routine operations in an imaging facility because the device provides:
   1. An indication of an individual's working habits
   2. An indication of working conditions in the facility
   3. A way for the employer to determine if radiation workers are actively engaged in performing a specific number of x-ray procedures during a given period
   A. 1 and 2 only
   B. 1 and 3 only
   C. 2 and 3 only
   D. 1, 2, and 3

4. The image densities cast by the filters in a film badge permit which of the following?
   A. Determination of the percentage of visible light emission
   B. Reuse of the radiographic film in the badge
   C. Estimation of the energy of the radiation reaching the badge
   D. Determination of the electrical discharge of the device

5. Which of the following personnel dosimeters allows a radiation worker to determine occupational exposure received as soon as a specific radiologic procedure is completed?
   A. Film badge
   B. OSL dosimeter
   C. Pocket dosimeter
   D. TLD

6. Which of the following instruments should be used in a laboratory to detect alpha and beta radiation and small amounts of other types of low-level radioactive contamination?
   A. Ionization chamber–type survey meter
   B. Proportional counter
   C. GM detector
   D. Pocket ionization chamber

7. Which of the following devices is used to measure the visible light emitted by the sensing material contained in the TLD *after* exposure to ionizing radiation and heating?
   A. Densitometer
   B. Laser
   C. Photomultiplier tube
   D. Sensitometer

8. In a health care facility, a radiographer's deep, eye, and shallow occupational exposures, as measured by an exposure monitor, may be found on the:
   A. Compliance report
   B. Quality assurance report
   C. Personnel monitoring report
   D. Worker's yearly evaluation

9. When the negatively and positively charged electrodes in the pocket ionization chamber are exposed to ionizing radiation, the mechanism does which of the following?
   A. It charges in direct proportion to the amount of radiation to which it has been exposed.
   B. It discharges in direct proportion to the amount of radiation to which it has been exposed.
   C. It heats the central electrode.
   D. It heats the quartz fiber indicator.

10. A densitometer is used to measure which of the following?
    A. Optical density
    B. The light emitted from sensing material of the TLD after exposure
    C. The luminescence from an OSL dosimeter
    D. Freed electrons and discharged electricity from all personnel dosimeters

11. Radiation survey instruments measure which of the following?
    1. The total quantity of electrical charge resulting from ionization of the gas
    2. The rate at which an electrical charge is produced
    3. Luminescence
    A. 1 and 2 only
    B. 1 and 3 only
    C. 2 and 3 only
    D. 1, 2, and 3

12. What do ionization chamber–type survey meters, proportional counters, and GM detectors have in common?
    A. They measure x-radiation and beta radiation only.
    B. They can be used to calibrate radiographic and fluoroscopic x-ray equipment.
    C. They are used to measure the radiation dose received outside protective barriers.
    D. Each contains a gas-filled chamber.

13. At the time of this printing, which of the following radiation monitors is *most commonly* used for monitoring occupational exposure in diagnostic imaging?
    A. Film badge
    B. Pocket ionization chamber
    C. TLD
    D. OSL

14. Which of the following are disadvantages of using a TLD as a personnel monitoring device?
    1. It can only be read once because the readout process destroys the stored information
    2. It is necessary to use calibrated dosimeters with TLD's
    3. The initial cost is higher than that for a film badge service
    4. Lithium fluoride is used as the sensing material in the TLD
    A. 1 and 2 only
    B. 1 and 3 only
    C. 1 and 4 only
    D. 1, 2, and 3 only

15. Before a pocket dosimeter is used to record radiation exposure, the quartz fiber indicator of the transparent reading scale should indicate which of the following?
    A. Zero (0)
    B. 100 mR
    C. 150 mR
    D. 200 mR

16. The OSL dosimeter uses:
    A. An Al_2O_3 detector
    B. LiF as a sensing material
    C. A miniature ionization chamber as a detector
    D. Radiation dosimetry film as a detector

17. A pocket ionization chamber resembles:
    A. A banana
    B. A compass
    C. An ordinary fountain pen
    D. A ruler

18. Monitoring companies send a control badge to health care facilities along with each batch of dosimeter badges. The control badge should be:
    A. Given as a monitor to a radiographer who loses his or her original badge
    B. Given as a second monitor to pregnant radiographer
    C. Given as a monitor to a radiographer working in the operating room
    D. Kept in a radiation-free area in the imaging facility

19. Dosimetry badge readings that exceed a trigger level set by the health care facility are investigated to:
    A. Ascertain the cause of the reading
    B. Determine whether wearing the badge was actually necessary
    C. Find grounds to fire the radiographer
    D. Increase the workload of the RSO to justify his or her position

20. The TLD readout process:
    A. Destroys the information stored in the TLD
    B. Saves the information stored in the TLD for future use
    C. Places the information in a computer
    D. Duplicates the stored information and sends a written report directly to the radiographer

21. An ionization chamber–type survey meter is also referred to as a:
    A. Cutie pie
    B. Flux capacitor
    C. Little rascal
    D. Warp drive

22. The increased sensitivity of the OSL dosimeter makes it ideal for monitoring employees working in low-radiation environments and for:
    A. Area monitoring of radioisotope storage facilities
    B. Monitoring of patients with a radioactive implant
    C. Monitoring of pregnant workers
    D. General patient monitoring

23. The RSO in a health care facility receives and reviews personnel monitoring reports to:
    A. Assess compliance with ALARA guidelines
    B. Assess compliance with National Academy of Sciences guidelines
    C. Gather information to compile a press report
    D. Meet guidelines established by the Health Insurance Portability and Accountability Act (HIPPA)

24. Wearing a personnel dosimeter in a consistent location is the responsibility of the:
    A. RSO
    B. Manager or director of the imaging department
    C. Chief radiologist
    D. Individual wearing the device

25. On termination of employment, a radiographer should receive a copy of:
    A. All personal health care records kept by the employer
    B. His or her occupational exposure report
    C. All employment records
    D. Incident reports in which the radiographer was involved

Exercise 4: True or False

Circle *T* if the statement is true; circle *F* if the statement is false.

1. T F Personnel dosimeters protect the wearer from exposure to ionizing radiation.
2. T F Wearing a personnel dosimeter in a consistent location is the responsibility of the individual wearing the device.
3. T F During special computed radiography, digital radiography, or conventional radiographic procedures, some health care facilities may prefer to have diagnostic imaging personnel wear two separate monitoring devices.
4. T F Cost is not a factor for health care facilities in selecting personnel dosimeters.
5. T F The film holder of a film badge dosimeter should be made of a plastic material of a high atomic number to filter low-energy x-radiation, gamma radiation, and beta radiation.
6. T F An ionization chamber-type survey meter cannot be used to measure exposures produced by typical diagnostic procedures because the exposure times are too long to permit the meter to respond.
7. T F A disadvantage of the OSL dosimeter is that occupational exposure cannot be established on the day of occurrence because the badge must be shipped to the monitoring company for reading and exposure determination.
8. T F Pocket ionization chambers require a special charging unit.
9. T F All radiation survey meters are equally sensitive in the detection of ionizing radiation.
10. T F The ionization survey–type meter is used for radiation protection surveys.

11. T F A film badge dosimeter may be worn for up to 1 year.

12. T F In health care facilities that have a well-structured radiation safety program, personnel monitoring reports are received and reviewed by the RSO.

13. T F A personnel dosimeter must be able to detect and record both small and large exposures in a consistent and reliable manner.

14. T F The filters in an OSL dosimeter are made of lead, potassium iodide, and zinc.

15. T F Ionizing radiation causes some of the physical properties of the LiF crystals in the TLD to undergo changes.

16. T F When changing employment, the radiation worker must convey the data pertinent to his or her accumulated permanent equivalent dose to the new employer so that this information can be placed on file.

17. T F Although an OSL dosimeter can work for up to 10 years, it commonly is worn for 2 years.

18. T F Pocket dosimeters provide no permanent legal record of exposure.

19. T F The primary advantage of a pocket ionization chamber is that it can provide an immediate exposure readout for radiation workers in high-exposure areas (e.g., a cardiac catheterization laboratory).

20. T F A TLD can be read numerous times.

21. T F Humidity, pressure, and normal temperature changes do not affect TLDs.

22. T F The GM detector is likely to saturate or jam when placed in a very-high–intensity radiation area, consequently giving a false reading.

23. T F Health care facilities must maintain a record of exposure recorded by personnel dosimeters as part of each radiation worker's employment record.

24. T F Area monitoring can be accomplished through the use of radiation survey instruments.

25. T F The image densities cast by the filters in the film badge allow estimation of the energy of the radiation reaching the badge.

Exercise 5: Fill in the Blank

Using the following Word Bank, fill in the blanks with the word or words that best complete the statements.

5	gestation	radiation output
40	inexpensive	reused
annually	ionization	second
charged	laser light	sensitive
contamination	legal	shallow
control	lost	sharply defined
cost-effective	medical physicists	thermoluminescent
deep	occupational	thyroid
densitometer	optically stimulated	trigger
electrometers	placement	usage
equivalent	plastic	worn
eyes	radiation-free	zero

1. When the personnel dosimeter is located at collar level, it provides a reading of approximate equivalent dose to the _____ gland and _____ of the occupationally exposed person.

2. Radiation survey instruments for area monitoring should be calibrated _____ to ensure accurate operation.

3. Personnel dosimeters include film badges, pocket _____ chambers, _____ _____ luminescence dosimeters, and _____ dosimeters.

4. Because many employees in a health care facility may be required to wear radiation monitors, they should be reasonably _____ to purchase and maintain.

5. A single exposure from a primary beam, such as would result if a radiographer inadvertently left the film badge on a table during an exposure, results in a _____ _____ image of the filters in the badge.

6. The control badge dosimeter should be kept in a _____ area in an imaging facility.

7. When changing employment, the radiation worker must convey those data pertinent to accumulated permanent _____ dose to the new employer.

8. Badge readings that exceed a _____ level set by the health care facility are investigated to ascertain the cause of the reading.

9. Before use each pocket dosimeter must be _____ to a predetermined voltage so that the quartz fiber indicator shows a _____ reading.

10. _____ _____ use ionization chambers connected to _____ to perform the standard measurements required by state, federal, and health care accreditation organizations for radiographic and fluoroscopic devices.

11. Radiation survey instruments are not all equally _____ in detecting ionizing radiation.

12. Because the GM detector allows for rapid monitoring, it can be used to locate a _____ radioactive source or low-level radioactive _____.

13. Ionization chambers can be used to measure the _____ _____ from both radiographic and fluoroscopic equipment.

14. Personnel monitoring ensures that _____ radiation exposure levels are kept well below the annual EfD limit.

15. The OSL dosimeter is "read out" by using _____ _____ at selected frequencies.

16. Pregnant diagnostic imaging personnel should be issued a _____ monitoring device to record the radiation dose to the abdomen during _____.

17. Monitoring reports list the _____, eye, and _____ occupational exposure of each person wearing the device in the facility as measured by the exposed monitor.

18. After a reading has been obtained, TLD crystals can be _____, making the device somewhat _____.

19. _____, badges indicate whether group badges were exposed in transit to or from a health care facility.

20. The front of the white paper packet of the OSL dosimeter may be color-coded to facilitate correct _____ and _____ of the badge on the body of occupationally exposed personnel.

21. The _____ is an instrument that measures occupational exposure by comparing optical densities of exposed film badges' (dosimetry) film.

22. A TLD is not effective as a monitoring device if it is not _____.

23. The film badge provides a permanent _____ record of personnel exposure.

24. The OSL dosimeter gives accurate readings as low as 1 mrem for x-rays and gamma ray photons with energies from _____ keV to greater than _____ MeV.

25. All components of an OSL dosimeter are sealed inside a tamperproof _____ blister packet.

Exercise 6: Labeling

Label the following illustration.

A. Pocket ionization chamber (pocket dosimeter)

1. _____

2. _____

Exercise 7: Short Answer

Answer the following questions by providing a short answer.

1. How do personnel dosimeters determine occupational exposure?

2. If an OSL dosimeter is used as a radiation monitor, why can occupational exposure not be determined on the day of occurrence?

3. What does an extremity dosimeter measure?

4. What information does the badge cover of an extremity monitor contain?

5. What is optical density?

6. List three radiation survey instruments that are used for area monitoring.

7. Where are proportional counters used? What do they detect?

8. List three disadvantages of a TLD.

9. What kind of detector is found in an OSL dosimeter?

10. What is the sensitivity range of radiation-dosimetry film used in a film badge dosimeter?

11. Why does a GM tube have a "check source" of a weak, long-lived radioisotope located on one side of its external surface?

12. When a protective lead apron is used during fluoroscopy or special procedures, why should the personnel dosimeter be worn outside the apron at collar level on the anterior surface of the body?

13. On a personnel monitoring report, what information is provided by the cumulative columns?

14. What does the letter *M* indicate when it appears under the current monitoring period or in the cumulative columns of a personnel monitoring report?

15. What must a radiation worker do when changing employment?

Exercise 8: General Discussion or Opinion Questions

The following questions are intended to allow students to express their knowledge and understanding of the subject matter, or to present a personal opinion. The questions may be used to stimulate class discussion. Because answers to these questions may vary, determination of an answer's acceptability is left to the discretion of the course instructor.

1. How can the GM detector be used as an area radiation survey instrument?

2. What responsibilities does a radiation safety officer fulfill in an imaging department?

3. Why is monitoring of radiation exposure important for occupationally exposed diagnostic imaging personnel?

4. How is the ionization chamber–type survey meter used for radiation protection surveys?

5. What requirements should radiation survey instruments used for area monitoring meet?

POST-TEST

The student should take this test after reading Chapter 4, finishing all accompanying textbook and workbook exercises, and completing any additional activities required by the course instructor. The student should complete the post-test with a score of 90% or higher before advancing to the next chapter. (Each of the following 20 questions or blanks is worth 5 points.) Score = _____ %

1. Some means of monitoring personnel exposure must be employed to ensure that occupational radiation exposure levels are kept well below the annual _____ dose limit.

2. Define the term *optically stimulated luminescence dosimeter*.

3. How can the working habits and working conditions of diagnostic imaging personnel be assessed over a designated period?

4. To meet state and federal regulations, _____ from personnel monitoring programs must be recorded accurately and maintained for review.

5. When a protective apron is not being used, where should a radiation worker wear a personnel monitoring device during routine computed radiography, digital radiography or conventional radiographic procedures, to approximate the location of maximal radiation dose to the thyroid and the head and neck?

6. Which of the following devices are used for personnel monitoring?
    1. OSL dosimeter
    2. TLD
    3. Ionization chamber-type survey meter (cutie pie)
   A. 1 and 2 only
   B. 1 and 3 only
   C. 2 and 3 only
   D. 1, 2, and 3

7. LiF functions as the sensing material in which of the following devices?
   A. Film badge
   B. OSL dosimeter
   C. Pocket dosimeter
   D. TLD

8. In a health care facility, where can a radiographer's deep, eye, and shallow occupational exposure as measured by an exposed monitor be found?

9. What instrument should be used to locate a lost radioactive source or to detect low-level radioactive contamination?

10. Before a pocket dosimeter is used to record radiation exposure, the quartz fiber indicator of the transparent reading scale should indicate a _____ reading.

11. In addition to a primary personnel dosimeter worn at collar level, pregnant imaging personnel should be issued a second monitoring device to record the radiation dose to the _____ during gestation to provide an estimate of the equivalent dose to the embryo-fetus.

12. When radiation workers change employment, what must they convey to the new employer?

_____

_____

13. Area monitoring can be accomplished through the use of radiation survey instruments. A simple detection system will indicate only the _____ or _____ of radiation, whereas a dosimeter system can quantitatively indicate both cumulative radiation _____ and radiation _____ _____.

14. Health care facilities must maintain a record of exposure recorded by personnel dosimeters as part of each radiation worker's _____ record.

15. When are radiation workers required to wear personnel monitoring devices?

_____

_____

16. It is recommended that an extremity dosimeter, or TLD ring badge, be worn by an imaging professional as a second monitor whenever procedures are performed that require the hands to be near the _____ x-ray beam.

17. In a health care facility who generally receives and reviews personnel monitoring reports?

_____

18. Although an OSL dosimeter can be worn for up to 1 year, it commonly is worn for _____ months.

19. What device is used to calibrate radiographic and fluoroscopic x-ray equipment?

_____

20. In diagnostic imaging, the increased sensitivity of the OSL dosimeter makes it ideal for monitoring employees working in low-radiation environments and for _____ workers.

5 Overview of Cell Biology

Chapter 5 covers basic concepts of cell biology. The chapter begins with a discussion of the cell and continues with other related topics, such as the chemical composition of cells. It includes a discussion of organic and inorganic compounds, cell structure, and cell division. This material lays the foundation for radiation biology, which is covered in subsequent chapters.

CHAPTER HIGHLIGHTS

- Cells are made of protoplasm, which consists of proteins, carbohydrates, lipids, nucleic acids, water, and mineral salts (electrolytes).
  - Proteins are essential to growth, construction, and repair of tissue; they may function as hormones and antibodies.
  - Carbohydrates provide fuel for cell metabolism.
  - Lipids act as a reservoir for long-term storage of energy, guard the body against the environment, and protect organs.
  - Nucleic acids (deoxyribonucleic acid [DNA] and ribonucleic acid [RNA]) carry genetic information necessary for cell replication.
  - Water constitutes the bulk of body weight, is essential for sustaining life, and serves as the transport medium for material the cell uses and eliminates.
  - Mineral salts maintain the correct portion of water in the cell, support cell function, aid in the conduction of nerve impulses, and prevent muscle cramping.
- Cells have several components:
  - The cell membrane surrounds the cell, functions as a barricade, and controls passage of water and other materials into and out of the cell.
  - Cytoplasm is the portion of a cell outside the nucleus in which all metabolic activity occurs.
  - The endoplasmic reticulum (ER) transports food and molecules from one part of the cell to another.
  - The Golgi apparatus unites large carbohydrate molecules with proteins to form glycoproteins.
  - Mitochondria contain enzymes that produce energy for cellular activity.
  - Lysosomes break down unwanted large molecules; they may rupture when exposed to radiation, resulting in cell death.
  - Ribosomes synthesize the various proteins that cells require.
  - The nucleus controls cell division, multiplication, and biochemical reactions.
- Somatic cells divide through the process of mitosis.
  - The cellular life cycle has four distinct phases of mitosis: pre–DNA synthesis, actual DNA synthesis, post–DNA manufacturing, and division.
  - Mitosis has four subphases: prophase, metaphase, anaphase, and telophase.
- Genetic cells divide through meiosis.
  - Meiosis is similar to mitosis except that no DNA replication occurs in telophase; the number of chromosomes in the daughter cell is reduced to half the number of chromosomes in the parent cell.
- The Human Genome Project has mapped the entire sequence of DNA base pairs on all 46 chromosomes.
  - There are 2.9 billion base pairs arranged into about 30,000 genes.

Exercise 1: Crossword Puzzle

Use the clues to complete the crossword puzzle.

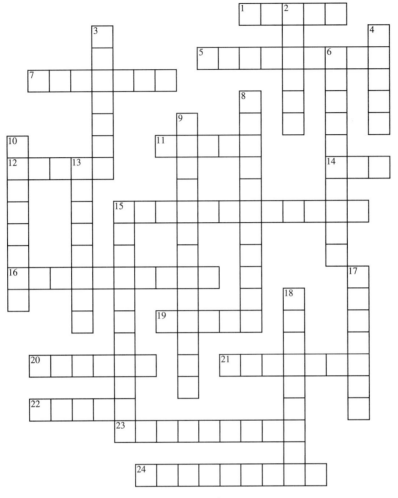

Down

2. Structural parts of cell membranes
3. Heart of the living cell
4. Chromosomal material
6. Protein molecules produced by specialized cells in the bone marrow in response to the presence of foreign antigens such as bacteria or viruses
8. Tiny rod-shaped bodies
9. Provide fuel for cell metabolism
10. Formed by combining amino acids into long chain-like molecular complexes
13. Small, insoluble, nonmembranous particles found in the cytoplasm
15. Coming from one zygote
17. Process by which somatic cells divide
18. Protein factories of the cell

Across

1. Units of a structure that can move, grow, react, protect themselves and repair damage, regulate life processes, and reproduce
5. Last phase of mitosis
7. Inorganic substance
11. Substance that aids in sustaining life
12. The steps in the DNA ladder
14. Female germ cells
15. Powerhouses of the cell
16. Unit formed from a nitrogen-containing organic base, a five-carbon sugar molecule (deoxyribose), and a phosphate molecule
19. Inorganic substances that keep the correct proportion of water in the cell
20. Basic constituent of all organic matter
21. Process of reduction cell division
22. Apparatus, bodies, or complex; minute vesicles that extend from the nucleus to the cell membrane and consists of tubes and a tiny sac located near the nucleus
23. Part of the cell that lies outside the nucleus
24. Phase of mitosis in which damage caused by radiation can be evaluated

Exercise 2: Matching

Match the following terms with their definitions or associated phrases.

1. _____ electrolytes
2. _____ antibodies
3. _____ human genome
4. _____ cytosine and thymine
5. _____ mapping
6. _____ enzymatic proteins
7. _____ cell division
8. _____ protoplasm
9. _____ anaphase
10. _____ protein synthesis
11. _____ hormones
12. _____ genes
13. _____ sodium and potassium
14. _____ cytoplasmic organelles
15. _____ carbohydrates
16. _____ adenine and guanine
17. _____ inorganic compounds
18. _____ deoxyribose
19. _____ lipids
20. _____ ribosomal RNA
21. _____ interphase
22. _____ nucleic acid
23. _____ organic compounds
24. _____ lysosomes
25. _____ cell membrane

A. Chemical building material for all living things
B. Made up of a molecule of glycerin and three molecules of fatty acid
C. Controls the cell's various physiologic activities
D. Mineral salts
E. Chemical secretions manufactured by various endocrine glands and carried by the bloodstream to influence the activities of other parts of the body
F. Process of locating and identifying genes in the genome
G. Protein production
H. Keep the correct proportion of water in the cell
I. A five-carbon sugar molecule
J. Compounds called *purines*
K. Compounds called *pyrimidines*
L. The total amount of genetic material (DNA) contained within the chromosomes of a human being
M. Protein molecules produced by specialized cells in the bone marrow called *B lymphocytes*
N. Multiplication process whereby one cell divides to form two or more cells
O. Saccharides
P. The phase of mitosis during which two chromatids repel each other and migrate along the mitotic spindle to opposite sides of the cell
Q. The frail, semipermeable, flexible structure that encases and surrounds the human cell and functions as a barricade to protect cellular contents from their outside environment; also controls the passage of water and other materials into and out of the cell
R. Segments of DNA that serve as the basic units of heredity
S. Small, pealike sacs or single-membrane spherical bodies that are of great importance for digestion within the cytoplasm
T. What all the miniature cellular components present in the cytoplasm of the cell are collectively called
U. Compounds that do not contain carbon
V. All carbon compounds, both natural and artificial
W. Functions to assist in the linking of messenger RNA to the ribosome to facilitate protein synthesis
X. Very large, complex macromolecules made up of nucleotides
Y. The period of cell growth that occurs before actual cell division

Exercise 3: Multiple Choice

Select the answer that *best* completes the following questions or statements.

1. In human beings, how many genes are contained in all 46 chromosomes?
   A. Approximately 300
   B. Approximately 3000
   C. Approximately 30,000
   D. Approximately 300,000

2. The nucleolus contains which of the following?
   A. Centrosomes and mitochondria
   B. Ribonucleic acid and proteins
   C. Ribosomes and Golgi bodies
   D. Lysosomes and endoplasmic reticulum

3. In the human cell, protein synthesis occurs in which of the following locations?
   A. Nucleus
   B. Mitochondria
   C. Ribosomes
   D. Endoplasmic reticulum

4. Interphase consists of which of the following phases?
   A. M, G_1, and S
   B. G_1, S, and G_2
   C. S, G_2, and M
   D. G_2, M, and G_1

5. Carbohydrates also may be referred to as:
   A. Lipids
   B. Nucleic acids
   C. Hormones
   D. Saccharides

6. DNA regulates cellular activity *indirectly* by reproducing itself in the form of _____ to carry genetic information from the cell nucleus to ribosomes located in the cytoplasm.
   A. Messenger DNA
   B. Messenger RNA
   C. Messenger REM
   D. Transfer RNA

7. Human cells contain which four major organic compounds?
   A. Nucleic acids, water, protein, and mineral salts
   B. Mineral salts, carbohydrates, lipids, and proteins
   C. Carbohydrates, lipids, nucleic acids, and water
   D. Proteins, carbohydrates, lipids, and nucleic acids

8. Which of the following is a process of reduction cell division?
   A. Mitosis
   B. Meiosis
   C. Molecular synthesis
   D. Amniocentesis

9. Which of the following cellular organelles function(s) as a cellular garbage disposal?
   A. Endoplasmic reticulum
   B. Mitochondria
   C. Lysosomes
   D. Ribosomes

10. Which of the following describes the nuclear envelope that separates the nucleus from other parts of the cell?
    A. Single membrane
    B. Double-walled membrane
    C. Triple-walled membrane
    D. Quadruple-walled membrane

11. Which of the following are functions of the cell membrane?
    1. Protecting the contents of the cell from the outside environment
    2. Controlling the passage of water and other materials into and out of the cell
    3. Allowing penetration by all substances into the cell

    A. 1 and 2 only
    B. 1 and 3 only
    C. 2 and 3 only
    D. 1, 2, and 3

12. Lipids are also referred to as:
    A. Amino acids
    B. Carbohydrates
    C. Fats
    D. Sugars

13. The primary energy source for the cell is:
    A. Amino acids
    B. Glucose
    C. Protein
    D. Phosphate

14. Cytosine bonds *only* with which of the following nitrogenous organic bases?
    A. Adenine
    B. Guanine
    C. Thymine
    D. Uracil

15. Which of the following statements is *not* true?
    A. Lysosomes are sometimes referred to as "suicide bags."
    B. Adenosine triphosphate (ATP) is essential for sustaining life.
    C. The Golgi apparatus or complex is the powerhouse of the cell.
    D. The nucleus is the "heart" of the cell.

16. When ionizing radiation is used to destroy malignant cells, an attempt is also made to spare healthy surrounding tissue. In radiation therapy this concept is referred to as a(n):
    A. Enzyme repair effect
    B. Therapeutic ratio
    C. Tissue tolerance effect
    D. Malignant cell annihilation effect

17. Twenty-two different _____ are involved in protein synthesis.
    A. Amino acids
    B. Antibodies
    C. Enzymes
    D. Hormones

18. The process of locating and identifying the genes in the human genome is called:
    A. Gene detecting
    B. Gene extrapolation
    C. Gene tracking
    D. Mapping

19. Approximately 80% to 85% of the weight of the human body is:
    A. Bone
    B. Fatlike substances
    C. Mineral salts
    D. Water

20. Meiosis is the process of:
    A. Converting inorganic substances into organic substances
    B. Identifying genes in the human genome
    C. Reduction cell division
    D. Repairing breaks in DNA

21. Water performs which of the following functions in the human body?
    1. Maintains a constant core temperature of 98.6° F (37° C)
    2. Regulates the concentration of dissolved substances
    3. Lubricates both the digestive system and the skeletal articulations (joints)
    A. 1 and 2 only
    B. 1 and 3 only
    C. 2 and 3 only
    D. 1, 2, and 3

22. Which of the following is of primary importance in maintaining adequate amounts of intracellular fluid?
    A. Deoxyribose
    B. Glucose
    C. Potassium
    D. Ribose

23. The S phase of mitosis is the:
    A. Pre–DNA synthesis phase
    B. Actual DNA synthesis period
    C. Post–DNA synthesis phase
    D. Phase when DNA synthesis multiplies by a factor of 4

24. When a cell divides, the genetic-containing material contracts into tiny rod-shaped bodies called:
    A. Golgi apparatus
    B. Chromosomes
    C. Mitochondria
    D. Nucleotides

25. Nitrogenous base pairs form the:
    A. Hormones needed by various endocrine glands in the body
    B. Mitotic spindle
    C. Steps, or rungs, of the DNA ladderlike structure
    D. Sugars the body needs for energy

Exercise 4: True or False

Circle *T* if the statement is true; circle *F* if the statement is false.

1. T F Cells are engaged in an ongoing process of obtaining energy and converting it to support their vital functions.

2. T F Depending on the cell type, water normally accounts for 25% to 35% of protoplasm.

3. T F Proper cell functioning depends on enzymes.

4. T F The skin is the body's initial barrier to any outside invasion by pathogens; however, once the skin has been penetrated, the body's primary defense mechanism against infection and disease is the hormones, which chemically attack any foreign invaders or antigens.

5. T F Lipids are organic macromolecules.

6. T F Nitrogen bonds attach the nitrogenous bases to each other, joining the two side rails of the DNA ladder.

7. T F A normal human being has 46 different chromosomes (23 pairs) in each somatic (nonreproductive) cell.

8. T F Genes control the formation of proteins in every cell through the intricate process of genetic coding.

9. T F All cellular metabolic functions occur in the nucleus.

10. T F Centrosomes are located in the center of the cell near the nucleus.

11. T F Different sequences of amino acids produce proteins with different functions.

12. T F Messenger RNA (mRNA) transfers its genetic code to another kind of RNA molecule, called *transfer RNA* (tRNA).

13. T F The cell membrane is a very thick structure that encases and surrounds the human cell.

14. T F Metabolism is the breaking down of large molecules into smaller ones.

15. T F Water is responsible for maintaining a constant body core temperature of 37° C.

16. T F Approximately 30,000 genes are contained in all 46 human chromosomes.

17. T F Radiation-induced damage to chromosomes may be evaluated during telophase.

18. T F Water lubricates the digestive system.

19. T F ATP is essential for sustaining life.

20. T F Sodium (Na) is the primary energy source for the human cell.

21. T F Genes control the formation of proteins in every living cell through the intricate process of genetic coding.

22. T F Cells are the basic units of all living matter, but they are not essential for life.

23. T F Proper cell function enables the body to maintain homeostasis, or equilibrium.

24. T F Lipids contain the most carbon of all the organic compounds.

25. T F Although carbohydrates are found throughout the body, they are most abundant in the spleen and nervous tissue.

Exercise 5: Fill in the Blank

Using the following Word Bank, fill in the blanks with the word or words that best complete the statement.

24	high	muscle
amino acids	homeostasis	nucleus
catalytic	hormones	osmotic
cell	liver	oxidative
DNA (term may be used more than once)	lysosomes	repair
	macromolecules	repair enzymes
electrolytes	metabolism (term may be used more than once)	replication
endoplasmic reticulum		ribosomes
fluid		salts
fraternal		

1. The _____ is the fundamental component of structure, development, growth, and life processes in the human body.

2. Proper cell function enables the body to maintain _____, or equilibrium.

3. The biomolecules that comprise protoplasm are formed from _____ elements.

4. Proteins are formed by combining _____ _____ into long, chainlike molecular complexes.

5. If radiation damage is excessive because of the delivered equivalent dose, the damage will be too severe for _____ _____ to have a positive effect.

6. _____ regulate body functions such as growth and development.

7. Although carbohydrates are found throughout the body, they are most abundant in the _____ and in _____ tissue.

8. The sequences of amino acids are determined by the order of the adenine-thymine and cytosine-guanine base pairs in the _____ macromolecule.

9. Maintaining the correct proportion of water in the cell maintains _____ pressure.

10. Dizygotic twins are also known as _____ twins.

11. Chromosomes are composed of _____.

12. Water tends to move across cell structures or membranes into areas with a _____ concentration of ions.

13. By balancing the concentration of potassium ions (as well as sodium and chlorine ions), the cell regulates the amount of _____ it contains.

14. _____ enables the cell to perform the vital functions of synthesizing proteins and producing energy.

15. Carbohydrates provide fuel for cell _____.
16. _____ synthesize the various proteins cells require.
17. Both the _____ and _____ capabilities of enzymes are vital to the survival of the cell.
18. Lipids are organic _____, large molecules built from smaller chemical structures.
19. By directing protein synthesis, the _____ plays an essential role in active transport, metabolism, growth, and heredity.
20. The _____ _____ transports food and molecules from one part of the cell to another.

21. Nucleic acids (DNA, RNA) carry genetic information necessary for cell _____.
22. _____ break down unwanted large molecules; they may rupture when exposed to radiation, resulting in cell death.
23. _____ metabolism is the breaking down of large molecules into smaller ones through the process of oxidation.
24. _____ are chemical compounds resulting from the interaction of an acid and a base.
25. Salts are sometimes referred to as _____.

Exercise 6: Labeling
Label the following illustrations and box.

A. Typical cell.

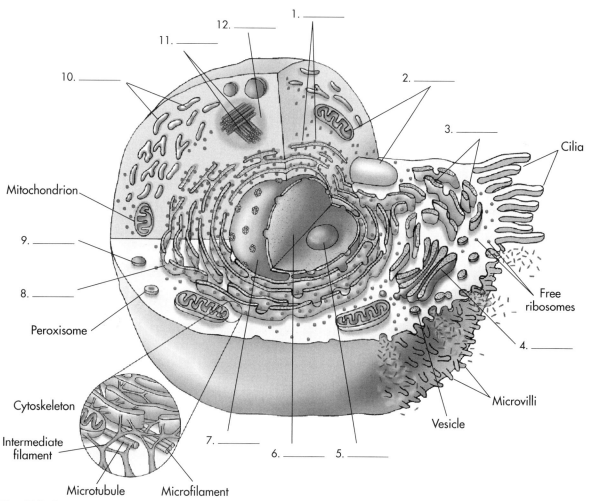

From Thibodeau A: *Anatomy and physiology*, ed 5, St Louis, 2003, Mosby.

B. Cellular life cycle.

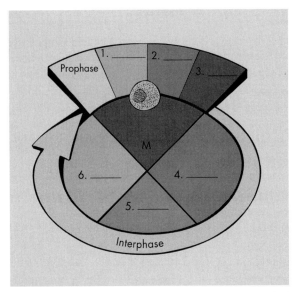

From Bushong SC: *Radiologic science for technologists: physics, biology and protection,* ed 9, St. Louis, 2008, Mosby Elsevier.

C. Summary of cell components

Title	Site	Activity
1. _____	Cytoplasm	Functions as a barricade to protect cellular contents from their environment and controls the passage of water and other materials into and out of the cell; performs many additional functions such as elimination of wastes and refining of material for energy through breakdown of the materials
2. _____	Cytoplasm	Enables the cell to communicate with the extracellular environment and transfers food from one part of the cell to another
3. _____	Cytoplasm	Unites large carbohydrate molecules and combines them with proteins to form glycoproteins and transports enzymes and hormones through the cell membrane so that they can exit the cell, enter the bloodstream, and be carried to areas of the body in which they are required
4. _____	Cytoplasm	Produce energy for cellular activity by breaking down nutrients through a process of oxidation
5. _____	Cytoplasm	Dispose of large particles such as bacteria and food as well as smaller particles; also contain hydrolytic enzymes that can break down and digest proteins, certain carbohydrates, and the cell itself if the lysosome's surrounding membrane breaks
6. _____	Cytoplasm	Manufacture the various proteins that cells require
7. _____	Cytoplasm	Believed to play some part in the formation of the mitotic spindle during cell division
8. _____	Nucleus	Contains the genetic material; controls cell division and multiplication and also biochemical reactions that occur within the living cell
9. _____	Nucleus	Holds a large amount of RNA

Exercise 7: Short Answer

Answer the following questions by providing a short answer.

1. What must the human body do to ensure efficient cell operation?

2. What is metabolism?

3. How are proteins formed? What determines the precise function of each protein molecule?

4. What functions do enzymatic proteins perform in the human body?

5. What are lipids? List six functions they perform for the human body.

6. What role do ribosomes play in the manufacture of protein by a cell?

7. Describe the function of water inside and outside the cells in the human body.

8. What does the nucleus in a human cell control?

9. List four distinct phases of the cellular life cycle.

10. How are a monosaccharide, a disaccharide, and a polysaccharide different?

11. List the four major classes of organic compounds found in the human body.

12. What is DNA?

13. What do structural proteins provide for the human body?

14. What is chromatin? What happens to this material when a cell divides?

15. What are hormones? What do the hormones that are produced in the thyroid gland control?

Exercise 8: General Discussion or Opinion Questions

The following questions are intended to allow students to express their knowledge and understanding of the subject matter or to present a personal opinion. The questions may be used to stimulate class discussion. Because answers to these questions may vary, determination of the answer's acceptability is left to the discretion of the course instructor.

1. Identify and describe the components of a typical human cell and discuss how cells perform many diverse functions for the body.

2. What is the Human Genome Project? What recent advances have been achieved through this project, and what challenges still remain?

3. Explain the process of mitosis.

4. What is the significance of inorganic and organic compounds in the human body?

5. What are enzymes, and what functions do they perform for the human body?

POST-TEST

The student should take this test after reading Chapter 5, finishing all accompanying textbook and workbook exercises, and completing any additional activities required by the course instructor. The student should complete the post-test with a score of 90% or higher before advancing to the next chapter. (Each of the following 20 questions or blanks is worth 5 points.) Score = _____ %

1. Cells are the basic units of all living _____ and are essential for life.

2. Proteins, carbohydrates, lipids, and nucleic acids are the four major classes of _____ compounds.

3. What type of enzymes can mend damaged molecules and therefore help the cell recover from a small amount of radiation-induced damage?
   _____

4. In a DNA macromolecule, adenine (A), cytosine (C), guanine (G), and thymine (T) are the four _____ organic bases.

5. Approximately 80% to 85% of the weight of the human body is _____.

6. Describe a DNA macromolecule.
   _____
   _____

7. What is the process of locating and identifying genes in the human genome called?
   _____

8. The large, double-membrane, oval or bean-shaped structures that function as the powerhouses of the cell are called:
   A. Endoplasmic reticulum
   B. Golgi apparatus
   C. Mitochondria
   D. Ribosomes

9. When somatic cells divide, they undergo:
   A. Centrosome removal
   B. Meiosis
   C. Mitosis
   D. Nuclear collapse

10. During which subphase of cell division can radiation-induced chromosomal damage be evaluated?
    _____

11. What function do ribosomes perform in the cell?
    _____

12. Approximately how many genes are contained in all 46 human chromosomes?
    _____

13. If exposure to ionizing radiation damages the components involved in molecular synthesis beyond repair, what will happen to the affected cells?

14. Protein synthesis involves _____ different amino acids.

15. What is formed from a nitrogen-containing organic base, a five-carbon sugar molecule, and a phosphate molecule?

16. What serves as a prototype for mRNA?

17. What is the protoplasm outside of the cell's nucleus called?

18. _____ is the period of cell growth that occurs before actual mitosis.

19. _____ act as a reservoir for long-term storage of energy, insulate and guard the body against the environment, and support and protect organs such as the eyes and kidneys.

20. What is the function of the cell membrane?

6 Molecular and Cellular Radiation Biology

Chapter 6 covers molecular and cellular radiation biology. The science of radiation biology encompasses the sequence of events occurring after the absorption of energy from ionizing radiation, the action of the living system to make up for the consequences of this energy assimilation, and the injury to the living system that may be produced. This chapter provides the reader with a basic knowledge of aspects of molecular and cellular radiation biology that are relevant to the subject of radiation protection. It also provides a foundation for an understanding of both early and late radiation effects on organ systems, which are covered in Chapters 7 and 8.

CHAPTER HIGHLIGHTS

- Linear energy transfer (LET)
  - LET is the average energy deposited per unit length of track by ionizing radiation as it passes through and interacts with a medium along its path.
  - It is described in units of kiloelectron volts (keV) per micron (1 micron [μm] = 10^{-6} m).
  - Low-LET radiation (x-rays and gamma rays) mainly causes indirect damage to biologic tissues, which usually can be reversed by repair enzymes.
  - High-LET radiation (alpha particles, ions of heavy nuclei, and low-energy neutrons) can cause irreparable damage to deoxyribonucleic acid (DNA) because multiple-strand breaks in DNA that cannot be undone by repair enzymes may result.
- Relative biologic effectiveness (RBE)
  - RBE for the type of radiation being used is the ratio of the dose of a reference radiation (conventionally 250-kVp x-rays) to the dose of radiation of the type in question that is necessary to produce the same biologic reaction in a given experiment; the reaction is produced by a dose of test radiation delivered under the same conditions.
  - As the LET of radiation increases, so do the biologic effects; RBE quantitatively describes this relative effect.
  - RBE describes the relative capabilities of radiation with differing LETs to produce a particular biologic reaction.
- Oxygen enhancement ratio (OER)
  - The OER is a comparative measure used to obtain the amount of cellular injury for a species of ionizing radiation.
- Radiation-induced damage is observed on the molecular, cellular, and organic levels.
- Radiation action on the cell is either direct or indirect, depending on the site of interaction.
  - Radiation action is direct when biologic damage occurs as a result of the ionization of atoms on DNA, causing them to become inactive or functionally altered.
  - Radiation action is indirect when effects are produced by reactive free radicals created by the interaction of radiation with water molecules; these unstable, highly reactive free radicals can cause substantial disruption to DNA molecules, which results in cell death.
  - High-LET radiation is more likely to cause biologic damage through direct action than is low-LET radiation.
  - Most x-ray damage to macromolecules is the result of indirect action.
  - Point mutations commonly occur with low-LET radiation and are reversible through the action of repair enzymes.
  - Double-strand breaks in DNA are associated with high-LET radiation, and repair of this type of damage is not likely to occur.
  - The target theory states that when cell DNA is directly or indirectly inactivated by exposure to radiation, the cell will die.
  - When a cell nucleus is significantly damaged by exposure to ionizing radiation, the cell can die or experience reproductive death, apoptosis, mitotic death, mitotic delay, interference with function, or chromosome breakage.
- The cell survival curve is used to display the radiosensitivity of a particular type of cell, which helps determine the types of cancer cells that will respond to radiation therapy.
- The law of Bergonié and Tribondeau states that the most pronounced radiation effects occur in cells having the least maturity and specialization, the greatest reproductive activity, and the longest mitotic phases.
  - The embryo-fetus is very susceptible to radiation damage, which can cause central nervous system (CNS) anomalies, microcephaly, and mental retardation.
  - Lymphocytes are the most radiosensitive blood cells, and when they are damaged, the body loses its natural ability to combat infection and becomes more susceptible to bacterial and viral antigens.
  - Human germ cells are relatively radiosensitive; temporary sterilization occurs at 2 Gy (200 rad); permanent sterilization occurs at 5 to 6 Gy (500 to 600 rad).

Exercise 1: Crossword Puzzle

Use the clues to complete the crossword puzzle.

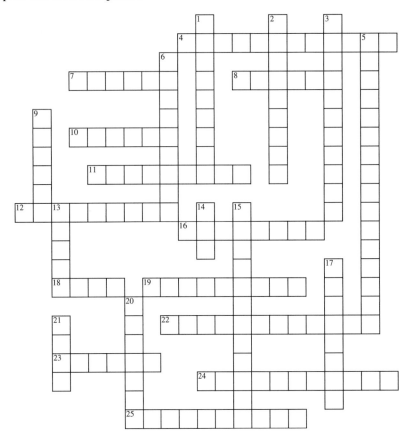

Down

1. Short-wavelength, high-energy waves emitted by the nuclei of radioactive substances.
2. Temporary condition that results from a single radiation dose of 2 Gy (200 rad) to the ovaries.
3. Process whereby single-chromosome breaks rejoin in their original configuration with no visible damage.
5. With reference to human cells and the impact of ionizing radiation on them, this is a factor that is variable.
6. Tentacle-like extensions from a nerve cell body that carry impulses toward the cell.
9. Type of water molecule that forms when hydrogen and hydroxyl ions recombine.
13. Particle composed of two protons and two neutrons.
14. Abbreviation for important factor used in assessing potential tissue and organ damage from exposure to ionizing radiation.
15. Scavenger type of white blood cells that fight bacteria.
17. Nonspecialized, rapidly dividing cells in the human body.
20. Type of delay that can be caused from exposing a cell to as little as 0.01 Gy (1 rad) of ionizing radiation just before it begins dividing.
21. What an ionized atom will not be able to do properly in molecules.

Across

4. May be used to explain cell death and nonfatal cell abnormalities caused by exposure to ionizing radiation.
7. Type of tissue considered relatively insensitive to radiation.
8. Action that is more likely to happen after exposure to high-LET radiation.
10. Enzymes that are capable of reversing damage from a single-strand break in a DNA macromolecule.
11. A nonmitotic, or nondivision, form of cell death that occurs when cells die without attempting division during the interphase portion of the cell life cycle.
12. Blood cells that initiate clotting and prevent hemorrhage.
16. What a therapeutic dose of ionizing radiation will cause in the blood count.
18. A long, single tentacle from a nerve cell body that carries impulses away from the cell.
19. Level on which biologic damage resulting from exposure to ionizing radiation begins.
22. Small head circumference.
23. Nerve cell.
24. Cross-link formed between two places in the same DNA strand.
25. A type of breakage that is a potential outcome when ionizing radiation interacts with a DNA macromolecule.

Exercise 2: Matching

Match the following terms with their definitions or associated phrases.

1. _____ direct action
2. _____ LET
3. _____ covalent cross-links
4. _____ radiation weighting factor (W_R)
5. _____ mutation
6. _____ cell survival curve
7. _____ indirect action
8. _____ OER
9. _____ apoptosis
10. _____ chromosome aberrations
11. _____ target theory
12. _____ RBE
13. _____ chromatid aberrations
14. _____ law of Bergonié and Tribondeau
15. _____ free radicals
16. _____ mitotic delay
17. _____ chromosome breakage
18. _____ R*
19. _____ molecular damage
20. _____ HO_2^*
21. _____ germ cells
22. _____ radiation biology
23. _____ hydrogen peroxide
24. _____ point mutation
25. _____ H* and OH*

A. Effects produced by reactive free radicals, which are created by the interaction of radiation with a water molecule.
B. The cell dies if inactivation of the master molecule occurs as a result of exposure to ionizing radiation.
C. Solitary atoms or most often a combination of atoms that behave as extremely reactive single entities as a result of the presence of unpaired electrons.
D. Used to calculate the equivalent dose to determine the ability of a dose of any kind of ionizing radiation to cause biologic damage.
E. Loss or change of a nitrogenous base in the DNA chain.
F. Lesions that result when irradiation occurs early in interphase, *before* DNA synthesis takes place.
G. Describes the relative capabilities of radiation with differing LETs to produce a particular biologic reaction.
H. Chemical unions created between atoms by the single sharing of one or more pairs of electrons.
I. Programmed cell death.
J. The radiosensitivity of cells is directly proportional to their reproductive activity and inversely proportional to their degree of differentiation.
K. Ratio of the radiation dose required to cause a particular biologic response of cells or organisms in an oxygen-deprived environment to the dose required to cause an identical response under normal oxygenated conditions.
L. Method of displaying the sensitivity of a particular type of cell to radiation.
M. Lesions that result when irradiation of individual chromatids occurs later in interphase, *after* DNA synthesis takes place.
N. Biologic damage that occurs as a result of ionization of atoms on master, or key, molecules (e.g., DNA), which causes these molecules to become inactive or functionally altered.
O. Average energy deposited per unit length of track.
P. The breaking of one or both of the sugar-phosphate chains of a DNA molecule, which can be caused by exposure of the molecule to ionizing radiation.
Q. Branch of biology concerned with the effects of ionizing radiation on living systems.
R. Injury on the molecular level resulting from exposure to ionizing radiation.
S. Female and male reproductive cells.
T. A hydrogen radical and a hydroxyl radical.
U. Genetic mutation in which the chromosome is not broken but the DNA within is damaged.
V. A hydroperoxyl radical.
W. An organic neutral free radical.
X. OH* + OH* = H_2O_2, a substance that is poisonous to the cell.
Y. Exposing a cell to as little as 0.01 Gy (1 rad) of ionizing radiation just before it begins dividing can result in failure of the cell to start dividing on time.

Exercise 3: Multiple Choice

Select the answer that *best* completes the following questions or statements.

1. Radiation damage is observed on which of the following three levels?
   A. Molecular, cellular, and inorganic
   B. Molecular, cellular, and organic
   C. Microscopic, molecular, and organic
   D. Organic, inorganic, and cellular

2. Molecular damage results in the formation of structurally:
   A. Changed molecules that permit cells to continue completing normal function
   B. Changed molecules that may impair cellular function
   C. Unchanged molecules that permit cells to continue functioning normally
   D. Unchanged molecules that may impair cellular function

3. According to the target theory, if only a few non-DNA cell molecules are destroyed by radiation exposure, the cell probably will:
   A. Not show any evidence of injury after irradiation
   B. Show evidence of injury after irradiation
   C. Show evidence of severe impairment after irradiation
   D. Die

4. Each cell's function is determined and defined by the structures of its constituent molecules. If these structures are altered by radiation exposure, the following may result:
   1. Disturbance of the cell's chemical balance
   2. Disturbance of cell operation
   3. Failure of the cell to perform normal tasks
   A. 1
   B. 1 and 2 only
   C. 1 and 3 only
   D. 1, 2, and 3

5. Chromosome aberrations happen when irradiation occurs:
   A. Early in interphase
   B. Late in prophase
   C. At the start of metaphase
   D. At the end of telophase

6. Which of the following are examples of distorted chromosomes?
   1. Anaphase bridges
   2. Dicentric chromosomes
   3. Ring chromosomes
   A. 1 and 2 only
   B. 1 and 3 only
   C. 2 and 3 only
   D. 1, 2, and 3

7. Which of the following may be used to explain cell death and nonfatal cell abnormalities caused by exposure to radiation?
   A. Covalent cross-linking
   B. Bergonié-Tribondeau law
   C. Programmed cell death
   D. Target theory

8. X-rays and gamma rays can be referred to as "streams of particles" because of a property known as:
   A. LET
   B. RBE
   C. Wave-particle duality
   D. Wave-particle fragmentation

9. The random interaction of x-rays with matter produces a variety of structural changes in biologic tissue, including:
   1. A single-strand break in one chromosome
   2. More than one break in the same chromosome
   3. Stickiness, or clumping together, of chromosomes
   A. 1 and 2 only
   B. 1 and 3 only
   C. 2 and 3 only
   D. 1, 2, and 3

10. Why are repair enzymes *usually* able to reverse the cellular damage generally caused by low-level ionizing radiation?
    A. Damage to DNA is sublethal.
    B. Irradiated cells are hypoxic.
    C. Only organic molecules are damaged.
    D. LET failed to occur.

11. What governs the radiation dose required to cause apoptosis?
    A. Changes in the cell protein content
    B. The phase of the cell cycle the individual cell is undergoing
    C. The radiosensitivity of the individual cell
    D. The number of cells irradiated

12. Which of the following describes the ratio of the radiation dose required to cause a particular biologic response of cells or organisms in an oxygen-deprived environment to the radiation dose required to cause an identical response under normal oxygenated conditions?
    A. OER
    B. Oxygen biologic effectiveness ratio
    C. Oxygen dose-response relationship
    D. Oxygen threshold ratio

13. Which of the following is a method of displaying the sensitivity of a particular type of cell to radiation?
    A. Cell survival curve
    B. Hypoxic cell measurement curve
    C. Radiolysis of water
    D. Radiation dose-response curve

14. Where are lymphocytes manufactured in the human body?
    A. Bone marrow
    B. Epithelial tissue
    C. Liver
    D. Pancreas

15. Which of the following defines the ratio of the dose of a reference radiation (conventionally 250 kVp x-rays) to the dose of radiation of the type in question that is necessary to produce the same biologic reaction in a given experiment?
    A. LET
    B. RBE
    C. W_R
    D. Low-level radiation effectiveness

16. A biologic reaction is produced by 6 Gy (600 rad) of a test radiation. It takes 36 Gy (3600 rad) of 250-kVp x-ray radiation to produce the same biologic reaction. What is the RBE of the test radiation?
    A. 3
    B. 6
    C. 9
    D. 12

17. A hydroperoxyl radical (HO_2^*) is formed when a hydrogen free radical (H^*) combines with:
    A. A hydrogen ion (H^+)
    B. A hydroxyl ion (OH^-)
    C. Molecular oxygen (O_2)
    D. Another hydrogen free radical (H^*)

18. LET is an important factor for:
    A. Assessing potential tissue and organ damage from exposure to ionizing radiation
    B. Assessing the characteristics of ionizing radiation (e.g., charge, mass, and energy)
    C. Determining the OER
    D. Removing electrons from tissue exposed to ionizing radiation

19. Because high-LET types of radiation deposit more energy per unit length of biologic tissue traversed, they are:
    A. More destructive to biologic matter than low-LET radiation
    B. Significantly less destructive to biologic matter than low-LET radiation
    C. Slightly less destructive to biologic matter than low-LET radiation
    D. Not comparable to low-LET radiation because they do not deposit any energy per unit length of biologic tissue traversed

20. Ring chromosomes, dicentric chromosomes, and anaphase bridges are examples of:
    A. Normal chromosomes
    B. Chromosomes about to divide
    C. Distorted chromosomes
    D. Chromosomes that carry appropriate genetic information

Exercise 4: True or False

Circle *T* if the statement is true; circle *F* if the statement is false.

1. T F The human body is a living system composed of large numbers of various types of cells, most of which cannot be damaged by radiation.

2. T F Biologic damage begins with the ionization produced by various types of radiation.

3. T F The characteristics of ionizing radiation (e.g., charge, mass, and energy) are exactly the same from one type of radiation to another.

4. T F LET is an important factor in the assessment of potential tissue and organ damage from exposure to ionizing radiation.

5. T F For radiation protection purposes, low-LET radiation is of the greatest concern when internal contamination is possible.

6. T F A positive water molecule (HOH^+) and a negative water molecule (HOH^-) are basically stable.

7. T F A few hundred centigray (cGy) (rad) of radiation can kill very sensitive cells such as lymphocytes or spermatogonia.

8. T F The embryo-fetus contains large numbers of mature, specialized cells and therefore is relatively radioresistant.

9. T F A blood count is a relatively insensitive test that is unable to indicate exposures of less than 10 cGy (10 rad).

10. T F Because the ovaries of young women are less sensitive than those of older women, a higher dose of radiation is required to cause sterility in young women.

11. T F Experimental data strongly indicate that ribonucleic acid (RNA) is the irreplaceable master, or key, molecule in the human cell.

12. T F Reproductive death generally results from exposure of cells to doses of ionizing radiation in the range of 1 to 10 Gy (100 to 1000 rad).

13. T F Ionizing radiation cannot adversely affect cell division.

14. T F Although it originally was applied only to germ cells, the law of Bergonié and Tribondeau is true for all types of cells in the human body.

15. T F LD 50/60 is more practical for human beings than LD 50/30.

16. T F If radiation damages the germ cells, the damage may be passed on to future generations in the form of genetic mutations.

17. T F The presence of free radicals in tissue does not affect the amount of biologic damage that results from irradiation.

18. T F X-ray photons may interact with but do not ionize water molecules in the human body.

19. T F Because hydrogen and hydroxyl ions usually recombine to form a normal water molecule, the existence of these ions as free agents in the human body is insignificant in terms of biologic damage.

20. T F A cell survival curve is constructed from data obtained from a series of experiments.

21. T F The human body is composed of different types of cells and tissues, all of which have the same degree of radiosensitivity.

22. T F In radiotherapy the presence of oxygen is not significant in terms of radiosensitivity.

23. T F The more mature and specialized in performing functions a cell is, the more sensitive it is to radiation.

24. T F Radiation affects primarily the stem cells of the hematopoietic (blood-forming) system.

25. T F The higher the radiation dose to the bone marrow, the more severe is the resulting cell depletion.

Exercise 5: Fill in the Blank

Using the following Word Bank, fill in the blanks with the word or words that best complete the statements.

0.25	energy	mitosis
2	gene	permanent
200	granulocytes	platelets
25	hydroxyl	radiosensitive
5	immature	(term may be used more than once)
500	infection	
6	insensitive	
600	internal	radiosensitivity
cellular	ionizing radiation	restored
charge	mass	sublethal
decrease	mental retardation	susceptible
dies	microcephaly	

1. Potentially harmful effects of ionizing radiation on living systems occur primarily at the _____ level.

2. X-ray and gamma-ray photons can impart _____ to orbital electrons in atoms if the photons happen to pass near the electrons.

3. Low-LET radiation generally causes _____ damage to DNA.

4. High-LET radiation includes particles with substantial _____ and _____.

5. High-LET radiation is of greatest concern when _____ contamination is possible.

6. The presence of oxygen in biologic tissues makes the damage produced by free radicals _____.

7. Approximately two thirds of all radiation-induced damage is ultimately believed to be caused by the _____ free radical (OH*).

8. _____ mutations could result from a single alteration along the sequence of nitrogenous bases in DNA.

9. _____ of the individual cell governs the dose required to cause apoptosis.

10. When _____ _____ interacts with cell atoms and molecules, the amount of radiation energy transferred (absorbed by the tissues) plays a major role in determining the extent of the biologic response.

11. Neutrophils, a type of white blood cell, play an important role in fighting _____.

12. Thrombocytes, or _____, initiate blood clotting and prevent hemorrhage.

13. _____ initially respond to radiation by increasing in number.

14. A therapeutic dose of radiation causes a _____ in the blood count.

15. Epithelial tissue has no blood vessels and regenerates through the process of _____.

16. Because the body constantly regenerates epithelial tissue, the cells comprising this tissue are highly _____.

17. Developing nerve cells in the embryo-fetus are more _____ than the mature nerve cells of adults.

18. Irradiation of the embryo may lead to CNS anomalies, _____, and _____.

19. Because mature spermatogonia are specialized and do not divide, they are relatively _____ to ionizing radiation.

20. Immature spermatogonia are unspecialized and divide rapidly; therefore these germ cells are extremely _____.

21. Nerve cells have a nucleus. If the nucleus of one of these cells is destroyed, the cell _____ and is never _____.

22. Temporary sterility usually results from a single dose of _____ Gy (_____ rad) to the ovaries.

23. Permanent sterilization occurs at _____ to _____ Gy (_____ to _____ rad).

24. The embryo-fetus, which has a large number of _____, nonspecialized cells, is much more _____ to radiation damage than is a child or an adult.

25. A whole-body radiation dose of _____ Gy (_____ rad) delivered within a few days produces a measurable hematologic depression.

Exercise 6: Labeling

Label the following illustrations and box.

A. Radiolysis of water.

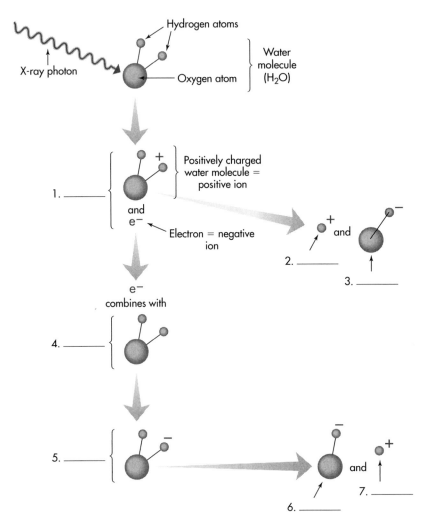

B. Indirect action of ionizing radiation on biologic molecules.

C. Examples of radiosensitive and radioinsensitive cells.

Radiosensitive Cells	Radioinsensitive Cells
1. _____	4. _____
2. _____	5. _____
3. _____	6. _____

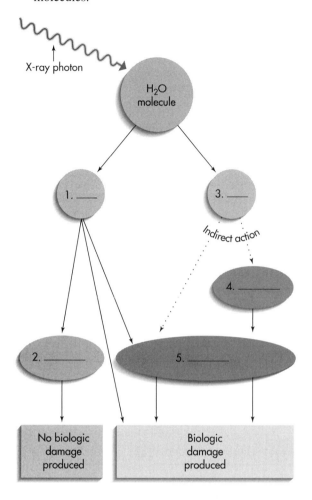

Exercise 7: Short Answer

Answer the following questions by providing a short answer.

1. How can high-energy particles, such as alpha and beta particles and protons, ionize atoms?

   _____

   _____

2. What determines the extent to which different radiation modalities transfer energy into biologic tissue?

   _____

   _____

3. In what unit of measure is LET generally described?

   _____

   _____

4. Why can repair enzymes usually reverse the cellular damage caused by low-LET radiation?

5. What are free radicals?

6. Which cells in the human body are classified as somatic cells?

7. How does oxygen enhance the effects of ionizing radiation in biologic tissue?

8. List seven ways damage to a cell's nucleus from ionizing radiation can reveal itself.

9. What is the difference between direct and indirect action of ionizing radiation on atoms or molecules in the human body?

10. If the nucleus in an adult human nerve cell is destroyed by exposure to ionizing radiation, what will happen to the cell?

11. How low a dose of ionizing radiation can cause menstrual irregularities, such as delay or suppression of menstruation?

12. List seven possible structural changes in biologic tissue caused by the random interaction of ionizing radiation with matter.

13. On what three levels is radiation damage observed?

14. When does ionizing radiation cause complete chromosome breakage?

15. How was the law of Bergonié and Tribondeau established? What does it state?

Exercise 8: General Discussion or Opinion Questions

The following questions are intended to allow students to express their knowledge and understanding of the subject matter or to present a personal opinion. The questions may be used to stimulate class discussion. Because answers to these questions may vary, determination of the answer's acceptability is left to the discretion of the course instructor.

1. What events can occur when an x-ray photon interacts with and ionizes a water molecule in the human body?

2. What are the possible consequences of radiation exposure to the embryo-fetus throughout the entire period of gestation?

3. Contrast the differences between high-LET radiation and low-LET radiation.

4. What are the possible effects of ionizing radiation on DNA?

5. What factors govern cell radiosensitivity? What are the effects of ionizing radiation on various types of cells in the human body?

POST-TEST

The student should take this test after reading Chapter 6, finishing all accompanying textbook and workbook exercises, and completing any additional activities required by the course instructor. The student should complete the post-test with a score of 90% or higher before advancing to the next chapter. (Each of the following 20 questions or blanks is worth 5 points.) Score = _____ %

1. A biologic reaction is produced by 7 Gy (700 rad) of a test radiation. It takes 21 Gy (2100 rad) of 250-kVp x-rays to produce the same biologic reaction. What is the RBE of the test radiation?

2. On which molecules in the human body does ionizing radiation most often act directly to produce molecular damage through an indirect action?

3. Radiosensitivity of the individual cell governs the radiation dose required to cause _____.

4. Define LET, and identify how it is described.

_____

_____

5. What is a comparative measure used to determine the amount of cellular injury for a species of ionizing radiation?

_____

6. The action of ionizing radiation is _____ when biologic damage occurs as a result of the ionization of atoms on DNA, causing them to become inactive or functionally altered.

7. Because even low doses of ionizing radiation from diagnostic imaging procedures can cause chromosomal damage, which of the following should be done whenever possible?
   A. Avoid all x-ray procedures until age 60
   B. Use a low kVp and high mAs technique
   C. Shield the reproductive organs
   D. Limit all radiographic procedures to just one projection per patient

8. Immature ova are:
   A. Somewhat radioinsensitive
   B. Significantly radioinsensitive
   C. Slightly radiosensitive
   D. Very radiosensitive

9. The _____ theory can be used to explain cell death and nonfatal cell abnormalities caused by exposure to radiation.

10. The action of ionizing radiation is _____ when effects are produced by reactive free radicals created by the interaction of radiation with water molecules; these unstable, highly reactive free radicals can cause substantial disruption of DNA molecules, which results in cell death.

11. What type of blood cells is classified as most radiosensitive?

_____

12. What law states that the most pronounced radiation effects occur in cells with the least maturity and specialization, the greatest reproductive activity, and the longest mitotic phases?

_____

13. Changes in genes caused by the loss of or a change in a base in the DNA chain are called _____.

14. What is a cell survival curve used to display?

_____

_____

15. An ionized atom will not _____ properly in molecules.

16. What can result within a few days, if an adult receives a whole-body ionizing radiation dose of 0.25 Gy (25 rad)?

_____

_____

17. If bone marrow cells have not been destroyed by exposure to ionizing radiation, they can _____ after a period of recovery.

18. A periodic _____ _____ is not recommended as a method of monitoring occupational radiation exposure because biologic damage already has been sustained when an irregularity is noted.

19. During the window of maximal sensitivity, a 0.1-Sv (10-rem) fetal equivalent dose is associated with as much as a 4% risk of _____ _____.

20. When does ionizing radiation cause complete chromosome breakage?

_____

_____

7 Early Radiation Effects on Organ Systems

Radiation-induced damage at the cellular level may lead to measurable somatic and genetic damage throughout the living organism. Chapter 7 focuses on early biologic responses demonstrated when the effects of radiation occur relatively soon after humans receive high doses of ionizing radiation. Numerous laboratory animal studies and data from observation of some human populations provide substantial evidence of the consequences of such responses. Although early effects are not common in diagnostic imaging, they are discussed in this chapter to provide the learner with a broader and more complete understanding of the impact of high radiation exposure on the human body.

CHAPTER HIGHLIGHTS

- Acute radiation syndrome (ARS) occurs when the whole body is exposed to 1 Gy (100 rad) of ionizing radiation.
    - ARS can manifest itself as hematopoietic syndrome, gastrointestinal syndrome, or cerebrovascular syndrome.
    - ARS has four major response stages: prodromal stage, latent period, manifest illness, and recovery or death.
- Lethal dose (LD) 50/30 signifies the whole-body dose of ionizing radiation that can be lethal to 50% of the exposed population within 30 days.
    - The LD in humans usually is given as LD 50/60 and is estimated to be 3 to 4 Gy (300 to 400 rad).
    - When cells are exposed to sublethal doses of ionizing radiation, repair and recovery are possible.
    - Surviving cells begin to repopulate.
    - Approximately 90% of radiation-induced damage may be repaired over time; 10% is irreparable.
- Early somatic effects occur within a short time after exposure to ionizing radiation.
    - These effects include nausea, fatigue, erythema, epilation, and blood and intestinal disorders.
- High radiation doses to any part of the human body can result in local tissue damage.
    - Cell death results from a substantial partial-body exposure, leading to atrophy of organs and tissues.
    - Depending on the type of cells involved and the dose of radiation received, recovery may be partial or complete or it may fail to occur, resulting in death of the irradiated biologic structure.
    - Factors such as radiosensitivity, reproductive characteristics, and growth rate govern organ and tissue response to radiation exposure.
- Many early radiologists and dentists developed radiodermatitis as a consequence of radiation exposure to the skin, eventually leading to the development of cancerous lesions.
    - Human skin consists of 3 layers and several accessory structures all of which are actively involved in the response of tissue to radiation exposure.
    - A single absorbed dose of 2 Gy (200 rad) can cause a radiation-induced skin erythema within 24 to 48 hours after irradiation.
    - High radiation doses can cause moist and then dry desquamation.
    - Moderate radiation doses can cause temporary hair loss, whereas large radiation doses can result in permanent hair loss.
    - Study of radiation therapy patients who received orthovoltage radiation therapy treatments provides significant evidence of skin damage caused by radiation exposure.
    - The use of high-level fluoroscopy for extended periods of time can result in radiation-induced skin injuries for patients.
- Human germ cells are relatively radiosensitive.
    - In males, a radiation dose of 0.1 Gy (10 rad) can depress the sperm population and possibly cause genetic mutations in future generations.
    - A radiation dose of 2 Gy (200 rad) may result in temporary sterility for up to a period of 1 year, and a dose of 5 to 6 Gy (500 to 600 rad) may result in permanent sterility.
    - In females, a gonadal dose of 0.1 Gy (10 rad) may delay or suppress menstruation. A single dose of 2 Gy (200 rad) to the ovaries can result in temporary sterility, and a dose of 5 to 6 Gy (500 to 600 rad) to the ovaries can result in permanent sterility.
    - Gonadal irradiation of the ovaries can result in genetic mutations that can be passed on to future generations. For this reason the ovaries should be shielded whenever possible during all imaging procedures.
- Periodic blood counts have been replaced by personnel dosimeters as a means to monitor occupational radiation exposure.
    - A measurable hematologic depression can be caused by a whole-body dose of radiation as low as 0.25 Gy (25 rad).
    - Lymphocytes are very radiosensitive. A radiation dose as low as 0.1 Gy (10 rad) can cause a decrease of these cells in the blood.

- A radiation dose of 0.5 Gy (50 rad) will cause a decrease in neutrophils, and a dose greater than 0.5 Gy (50 rad) can cause a decrease in the number of thrombocytes (platelets).
- A depletion of cells that protect the body against disease results in the body losing its ability to fight infection.
■ Mapping of chromosomes is called *karyotyping*.
- Karyotyping is done during metaphase, when each chromosome can be individually demonstrated and radiation-induced chromosome and chromatid aberrations can be observed.
- Chromosomal damage can be caused by both low and high radiation doses.
- Chromosomal aberrations have been observed in individuals after completion of imaging procedures in which a high radiation dose rate was used.

Exercise 1: Crossword Puzzle

Use the clues to complete the crossword puzzle.

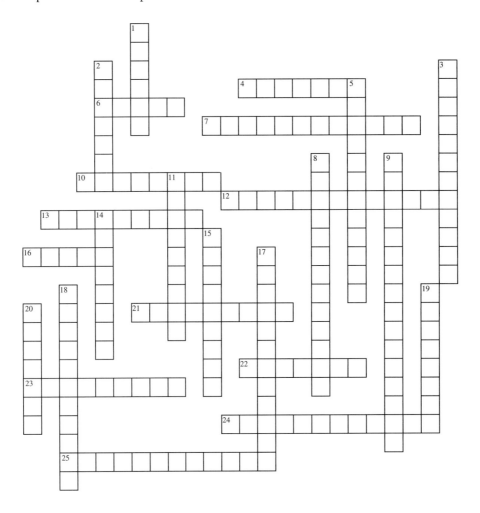

Down

1. Anatomic part of the human male that contains both mature and immature spermatogonia.
2. Ovarian stem cells that multiply to millions of cells only during fetal development, before birth, and then steadily decline in number throughout life.
3. Type of white blood cells that act as scavengers to fight bacteria.
5. The study of cell genetics with emphasis on cell chromosomes.
8. Term that is synonymous with *bone marrow syndrome*.
9. The workers and firefighters at Chernobyl are examples of humans who died as a result of this dose-related syndrome that occurs as part of the acute radiation syndrome.
11. Outer layer of the skin.
14. Diffused redness that appears over an area of skin after irradiation.
15. What LD 50/30, LD 50/60, and LD 100/60 are used to measure.

17. Red blood cells that initiate blood clotting and prevent hemorrhage.
18. White blood cells that play an active role in producing immunity for the body by producing antibodies to combat disease.
19. Medical term that means a collection of symptoms.
20. Process of shrinking of organs and tissues.

Across

4. Term used to describe poorly oxygenated cells.
6. X-rays in the energy range of 10 to 20 kVp that were once used to treat skin diseases such as ringworm.
7. Shedding of the outer layer of skin.
10. Stage of illness in acute radiation syndrome when symptoms that were not visible in the week preceding this stage become visible.
12. Term that is synonymous with nonstochastic.
13. Chromosomes having two centromeres.
16. Effects of radiation not common in diagnostic imaging.
21. Loss of hair.
22. Boston dentist who began investigating the hazards of radiation exposure and became the first known advocate of radiation protection.
23. Synonymous term used to describe the initial stage of ARS.
24. Type of radiation therapy treatment that provides significant evidence of skin damage.
25. Red blood cells that through their hemoglobin carry oxygen from the lungs to all body tissue and cells as blood circulates.

Exercise 2: Matching

Match the following terms with their definitions or associated phrases.

1. _____ biologic dosimetry
2. _____ skin
3. _____ LD 50/30
4. _____ ovulation
5. _____ mature spermatogonia
6. _____ dermis
7. _____ bone marrow syndrome
8. _____ Marshall Islanders
9. _____ leukopenia
10. _____ decrease
11. _____ epilation
12. _____ necrosis, or death
13. _____ cerebrovascular syndrome
14. _____ deterministic effects
15. _____ ARS
16. _____ oocytes
17. _____ 1920s and 1930s

A. Specialized, nondividing cells that are relatively radioresistant.
B. Early nonstochastic somatic effects that result from high doses of radiation.
C. A single precursor cell from which all cells of the hematopoietic system develop.
D. Form of ARS that occurs when humans receive whole-body doses of ionizing radiation ranging from 1 to 10 Gy (100 to 1000 rad).
E. Functions as an ongoing regeneration system for the human body; is relatively radiosensitive.
F. Immature female germ cells.
G. Population inadvertently subjected to high levels of fallout during an atomic bomb test in 1954.
H. Result when an organ or tissue fails to recover from radiation exposure.
I. What radiation exposure causes the number of red cells, white cells, and platelets in the circulating blood to do.
J. An abnormal decrease in white blood corpuscles, usually below 5000/mm^3.
K. Period during the female menstrual cycle when a mature follicle releases an ovum.
L. Form of ARS that appears at a threshold dose of approximately 6 Gy (600 rad).
M. Whole-body dose of ionizing radiation that can be lethal to 50% of the exposed population within 30 days.
N. Middle layer of skin.
O. A method of dose assessment in which biologic markers or effects of radiation exposure are measured and the dose to the organism is inferred from previously established dose-effect relationships.
P. Radiation sickness that occurs in human beings after whole-body reception of large doses of ionizing radiation (1 Gy [100 rad] or more) delivered over a short time.
Q. Period of time when periodic blood counts were the only means of radiation exposure monitoring for radiation workers engaged in radiologic practices.

18. _____ pluripotential stem cell
19. _____ prodromal stage
20. _____ gastrointestinal syndrome
21. _____ manifest illness
22. _____ chromosome aberrations
23. _____ latent period
24. _____ anemia
25. _____ burns

R. A decrease in the number of blood cells in the circulating blood can result in a lack of vitality and this condition.
S. The period after the initial stage of ARS during which no visible effects or symptoms of radiation exposure occur.
T. Thermal trauma.
U. The stage of ARS in which symptoms become visible.
V. The first stage of ARS, which occurs within hours after a whole-body absorbed dose of 1 Gy (100 rad) or more; it is characterized by nausea, vomiting, diarrhea, fatigue, and leukopenia.
W. Deviation from normal development or growth.
X. Form of ARS that results when the central nervous system and the cardiovascular system receive ionizing radiation doses of 50 Gy (5000 rad) or more.
Y. Alopecia.

Exercise 3: Multiple Choice

Select the answer that *best* completes the following questions or statements.

1. When biologic effects from ionizing radiation demonstrate the existence of a threshold and the severity of that damage *increases* as a consequence of increased absorbed dose, the events are considered:
   A. Deterministic
   B. Probabilistic
   C. Stochastic
   D. Unimportant

2. Approximately what percent of the human body's surface skin cells are replaced daily by stem cells from an underlying basal layer?
   A. 2%
   B. 12%
   C. 35%
   D. 50%

3. A cytogenetic analysis of chromosomes may be accomplished through the use of a chromosome map. This may is called a:
   A. Chromosomogram
   B. Karyograph
   C. Karyotype
   D. Photocytogenetic plot

4. During the age of approximately 12 to 50, how many mature ova will a female produce?
   A. 50 to 100
   B. 100 to 200
   C. 300 to 400
   D. 400 to 500

5. Which of the following are parts of the hematopoietic system?
   1. Bone marrow
   2. Circulating blood
   3. Lymphoid organs
   A. 1 and 2 only
   B. 1 and 3 only
   C. 2 and 3 only
   D. 1, 2, and 3

6. Many early radiologists and dentists developed a reddening of the skin caused by exposure to ionizing radiation. This condition is called:
   A. Dermabrerration
   B. Desquamation
   C. Epidermatitis
   D. Radiodermatitis

7. Which of the following measures of lethality may be a more relevant indicator of outcome for humans?
   A. LD 10/30
   B. LD 50/30
   C. LD 50/60
   D. LD 100/60

8. On which of the following factors does somatic or genetic radiation-induced damage depend?
   1. The amount of body area exposed
   2. The quantity of ionizing radiation to which the subject is exposed
   3. The specific parts of the body exposed
   A. 1 only
   B. 2 only
   C. 3 only
   D. 1, 2, and 3

9. In humans with the gastrointestinal form of ARS, the part of the body *most* severely affected is the:
   A. Brain
   B. Heart
   C. Large intestine
   D. Small intestine

10. Which of the following occurs in humans after whole-body reception of large doses of ionizing radiation delivered over a short period of time?
    A. Acute radiation syndrome
    B. Hypertension
    C. Multiple sclerosis
    D. Tuberculosis

11. The use of high-level fluoroscopy for extended periods of time can result in:
    A. A significant reduction in radiation-induced skin injuries for patients
    B. Minimal total-body radiation exposure for patients
    C. Radiation-induced skin injuries for patients
    D. The need for all patients to have periodic blood counts to monitor radiation dose received

12. What do the atomic bomb survivors of Hiroshima and Nagasaki, the Marshall Islanders inadvertently subjected to high levels of fallout during an atomic bomb test in 1954, and the nuclear radiation victims of the 1986 Chernobyl disaster have in common?
    A. All were exposed to low-level ionizing radiation.
    B. All were exposed to high levels of ionizing radiation, but no group members experienced any appreciable bodily damage.
    C. All were exposed to doses of ionizing radiation sufficient to cause ARS in many group members.
    D. These groups have nothing in common.

13. Which of the following factors govern organ and tissue response to radiation exposure?
    1. Growth rate
    2. Radiosensitivity
    3. Reproductive characteristics
    A. 1 and 2 only
    B. 1 and 3 only
    C. 2 and 3 only
    D. 1, 2, and 3

14. Which of the following does *not* cause early (acute) deterministic somatic effects of ionizing radiation?
    A. Doses greater than 3 Gy (300 rad)
    B. Doses greater than 6 Gy (600 rad)
    C. Doses resulting from atomic bomb detonation
    D. Doses encountered in diagnostic radiology

15. The hematopoietic, gastrointestinal, and cerebrovascular syndromes are three separate dose-related syndromes that are part of the:
    A. Bone marrow syndrome
    B. Cytogenetic syndrome
    C. Prodromal syndrome
    D. Total-body syndrome

16. Without effective physical monitoring devices, what biologic criteria would play an important role in the identification of radiation casualties during the first 2 days after a nuclear disaster?
    A. Coma
    B. Edema in the cranial vault
    C. Meningitis
    D. Occurrence of nausea and vomiting

17. Without medical support, the LD 50/30 for adult humans is estimated to be:
    A. 1.0 to 2.0 Gy (100 to 200 rad)
    B. 2.0 to 3.0 Gy (200 to 300 rad)
    C. 3.0 to 4.0 Gy (300 to 400 rad)
    D. 4.0 to 5.0 Gy (400 to 500 rad)

18. Infection, hemorrhage, and cardiovascular collapse are symptoms that can occur as part of acute radiation syndrome during the:
    1. Initial stage
    2. Latent period
    3. Stage called *manifest illness*
    A. 1 only
    B. 2 only
    C. 3 only
    D. 1, 2, and 3

19. Which of the following local tissues will experience immediate consequences from high radiation doses?
    1. Bone marrow
    2. Male and female reproductive organs
    3. Skin
    A. 1 and 2 only
    B. 1 and 3 only
    C. 2 and 3 only
    D. 1, 2, and 3

20. Imaging procedures generally result in:
    A. Relatively low doses of gonadal radiation for the patient and for imaging personnel
    B. Moderate doses of gonadal radiation for the patient and for imaging personnel
    C. High doses of gonadal radiation for the patient and for imaging personnel
    D. Relatively low doses of gonadal radiation for the patient and very high gonadal doses for imaging personnel

21. Which of the following are accessory structures of the skin?
    1. Hair follicles
    2. Sebaceous glands
    3. Sweat glands
    A. 1 and 2 only
    B. 1 and 3 only
    C. 2 and 3 only
    D. 1, 2, and 3

22. When cells are exposed to sublethal doses of ionizing radiation, repair and recovery may occur because cells:
    A. Are completely insensitive to radiation exposure
    B. Contain a repair mechanism inherent in their biochemistry (repair enzymes)
    C. Exposed to sublethal doses become hypoxic and recover more efficiently
    D. Mutate and become radioresistant

23. The testes of the human male and the ovaries of the female do *not* respond the same way to irradiation because:
    A. The oogonia, the ovarian stem cells of the female, constantly reproduce throughout life
    B. There is a difference in the way in which male and female germ cells are produced and progress from elementary stem cells to mature cells
    C. The oogonia become encapsulated by numerous primordial follicles during development
    D. The spermatogonia of the male never mature

24. When are the ovaries of the human *most* radiosensitive?
    A. During the fetal stages of life and during early childhood
    B. After puberty and the onset of menstruation
    C. From 20 to 30 years of age
    D. During pregnancy

25. ARS is actually a collection of symptoms associated with:
    A. Exposure to low-level radiation
    B. Exposure to moderate-level radiation
    C. Exposure to high-level radiation
    D. Exposure to nonionizing radiation

Exercise 4: True or False

Circle *T* if the statement is true; circle *F* if the statement is false.

1. T F Current radiation protection programs rely on hematologic depression as a means for monitoring imaging personnel to assess if they have sustained any degree of radiation damage from occupational exposure.

2. T F If cells that are needed to clot blood are depleted, the risk of hemorrhage decreases.

3. T F Telophase is the phase of cell division in which chromosomal damage caused by radiation exposure can be evaluated.

4. T F If the effects of ionizing radiation are cell-killing and directly related to the dose received, they are called *nonstochastic (deterministic) somatic effects*.

5. T F A person who has received a radiation exposure sufficient to cause radiation sickness will experience the initial stage of the syndrome within hours after the whole-body absorbed dose. After this stage, no visible symptoms occur for about 1 week.

6. T F Radiation exposure causes an increase in the number of red cells, white cells, and platelets in the circulating blood.

7. T F The LD 50/30 for adult human beings is estimated to be 8 to 9 Gy (800 to 900 rad).

8. T F The Japanese atomic bomb survivors of Hiroshima and Nagasaki are examples of a human population with ARS as a consequence of war.

9. T F Radiation therapy patients who received orthovoltage radiation therapy treatments provide significant evidence of skin damage caused by radiation exposure.

10. T F Early somatic effects occur within a long period of time after exposure to ionizing radiation.

11. T F Ionizing radiation produces the greatest amount of biologic damage to the human body when a small dose of sparsely ionizing (low-LET) radiation is delivered to a small or radiosensitive area of the body.

12. T F ARS actually is a collection of symptoms associated with low-LET radiation exposure.

13. T F Intestinal disorders are caused by radiation damage to the sensitive epithelial tissue lining the intestines.

14. T F Radiation doses ranging from 1 to 10 Gy (100 to 1000 rad) produce an increase in the number of bone marrow stem cells.

15. T F In the human female a gonadal dose of 0.1 Gy (10 rad) may delay or suppress menstruation.

16. T F Whole-body equivalent doses greater than 1 Gy (100 rad) are considered fatal regardless of medical treatment.

17. T F Moderate radiation doses can cause temporary hair loss, and large radiation doses can result in permanent hair loss.

18. T F Chromosomal damage can be caused by both low and high radiation doses.

19. T F Karyotyping is done during anaphase, when each chromosome can be individually demonstrated and radiation-induced chromosome and chromatid aberrations can be observed.

20. T F As a result of the effects of the atomic bomb in Japan and the nuclear accident at Chernobyl, the medical community has recognized the need for a thorough understanding of ARS and appropriate medical support of victims.

21. T F The massive explosion at the Chernobyl nuclear power plant on April 26, 1986 ejected several tons of burning graphite, uranium dioxide fuel, and other contaminants (e.g., cesium-137, iodine-131, and plutonium-239) vertically into the atmosphere in a 3-mile-high, radioactive plume of intense heat.

22. T F LD 50/30 for humans may be more accurate than LD 50/60.

23. T F The workers and firefighters at Chernobyl are examples of humans who died as a result of the gastrointestinal syndrome.

24. T F Only some layers of the skin and its accessory structures are actively involved in the response of the tissue to radiation exposure.

25. T F Highly specialized, nondividing cells in the circulating blood with the exception of lymphocytes are relatively insensitive to radiation.

Exercise 5: Fill in the Blank

Using the following Word Bank, fill in the blanks with the word or words that best complete the statements.

0.25 (25)	direct action	photograph
1 (100)	early	photomicrograph
2 (200)	functional	platelets
10	high	radiation sickness
20	impaired fertility	radiosensitive
anemia	indirect action	repair
atrophy	ionizing radiation	repopulation
biologic criteria	late	substantial dose
chromosomal abnormalities	menstruation	William Herbert Rollins
death	neutrophils	

1. A _____ _____ of ionizing radiation is required to produce biologic effects soon after irradiation.

2. Acute radiation syndrome (ARS) occurs when the whole body is exposed to _____ Gy (_____ rad) or more.

3. _____ _____ is another term for *acute radiation syndrome* (ARS).

4. Depending on the length of time from the moment of irradiation to the first appearance of symptoms of radiation damage, the effects are classified as either _____ or _____ somatic effects.

5. Because the number of _____ decreases with loss of bone marrow function, the body loses a corresponding amount of its blood-clotting ability.

6. During the accident at the Chernobyl nuclear power plant in 1986, dose assessment was determined from _____ _____.

7. Whole-body radiation doses greater than 6 Gy (600 rad) may cause the _____ of the entire population in 30 days without medical support.

8. When the processes of _____ and _____ work together, they aid in healing the body from radiation injury and promote recovery.

9. The amount of _____ damage sustained determines an organ's potential for recovery.

10. A response in biologic tissue can occur when any part of the human body receives a _____ radiation dose.

11. Safety practices such as wearing radiopaque glasses, enclosing the x-ray tube in a protective housing, and irradiating only areas of interest on the patient were recommendations made by _____.

12. A single absorbed dose of _____ Gy (_____ rad) can cause a radiation-induced skin erythema within 24 to 48 hours after irradiation.

13. During cardiovascular or therapeutic interventional procedures that use high-level fluoroscopy for extended periods of time, patient exposure rates have been estimated to range from _____ to _____ R per minute and sometimes even greater.

14. Human germ cells are relatively _____.

15. If an ovum is not fertilized by a male sperm, it will be lost during _____ and not replaced.

16. High radiation doses to the testes can result in _____.

17. Because any dose of radiation to the gonads could cause _____ _____, the testes should be protected with lead shielding whenever possible.

18. In the years when periodic blood counts were used for radiation monitoring purposes, a whole-body dose as low as _____ Gy (_____ rad) would produce a measurable hematologic depression.

19. A decrease in the number of red blood cells in the circulating blood can result in a lack of vitality and a condition known as _____.

20. Most chromosomal damage results from the process of _____ _____ of ionizing radiation on vital biologic macromolecules.

21. A chromosome may consist of a _____, or _____.

22. Only a very small percent of damage that causes chromosome breakage occurs from _____ _____ of ionizing radiation on a macromolecule such as DNA.

23. Almost every type of chromosome aberration can be caused by exposure to _____ _____.

24. A radiation dose of 0.5 Gy (50 rad) will cause a decrease in _____.

25. For the female, _____ _____ may not be the only consequence of gonadal irradiation.

Exercise 6: Labeling

Label the following table and illustrations.

A. Overview of acute radiation lethality.

Stage	Dose (Gy [rad])	Average Survival Time	Signs and Symptoms
1. _____	1 (100)	—	Nausea, vomiting, diarrhea, fatigue, leukopenia
2. _____	1-100 (100-10,000)	—	None
3. _____	1-10 (100-1000)	6-8 wk (doses over 2 Gy)	Nausea; vomiting; diarrhea; decrease in number of red blood cells, white blood cells, and platelets in the circulating blood; hemorrhage; infection
4. _____	6-10 (600-1000)	3-10 days	Severe nausea, vomiting, diarrhea, fever, fatigue, loss of appetite, lethargy, anemia, leukopenia, hemorrhage, infection, electrolytic imbalance, and emaciation
5. _____	50 and above (5000 and above)	Several hours to 2 or 3 days	Same as hematopoietic and gastrointestinal, excessive nervousness, confusion, lack of coordination, loss of vision, a burning sensation of the skin, loss of consciousness, disorientation, shock, periods of agitation alternating with stupor, edema, loss of equilibrium, meningitis, prostration, respiratory distress, vasculitis, coma

B. Development of the germ cell from stem cell phase to the mature cell.

Male:

1._____ 2._____ 3._____ 4._____

Female:

1._____ 2._____ 3._____ 4._____

C. Progressive development of various cells from a single pluripotential stem cell.

Exercise 7: Short Answer

Answer the following questions by providing a short answer.

1. What has provided substantial evidence of the consequences of early biologic responses to high doses of ionizing radiation?

   _____

   _____

2. During the explosion at the Chernobyl nuclear power plant in 1986, what are some of the radioactive materials that were ejected vertically into the atmosphere in a 3-mile-high radioactive plume of intense heat?

   _____

   _____

3. Name the four stages of ARS.

4. Name the three forms of ARS.

5. What happens to the human body when cells of the lymphatic system are damaged by radiation exposure?

6. Why is a bone marrow transplant not an absolute cure for patients with the hematopoietic syndrome?

7. What are some symptoms of the cerebrovascular syndrome?

8. To what have the techniques used to study and observe the chromosomes of each human cell contributed?

9. If there is a decrease in the number of highly radiosensitive stem cells in bone marrow as a consequence of irradiation, how will this decrease manifest itself?

10. If both oxygenated and hypoxic cells receive a comparable dose of low-LET radiation, what impact will the radiation dose have on each of these types of cells?

11. What are the most important measures used to quantify human radiation lethality?

12. When cells of the lymphatic system are damaged by ionizing radiation, what is the consequence to the human body?

13. When shedding of the outer layer of skin occurs after reception of higher radiation doses, how does it generally manifest itself?

14. What was the goal of orthovoltage radiation therapy treatment?

15. Why is LD 50/60 a more relevant indicator of outcome than LD 50/30 for humans who have received a substantial dose of ionizing radiation?

Exercise 8: General Discussion or Opinion Questions

The following questions are intended to allow students to express their knowledge and understanding of the subject matter or to present a personal opinion. The questions may be used to stimulate class discussion. Because answers to these questions may vary, determination of the answer's acceptability is left to the discretion of the course instructor.

1. What has been the mental and physical impact on the exposed population of the 1986 accident at the Chernobyl nuclear power plant?

2. What knowledge of early effects of high-dose radiation exposure has been gained from pioneers in the radiation field and from exposed populations?

3. How do human male and female germ cells differ in their development?

4. What type of local tissue damage can occur from high radiation exposure?

5. What is the potential for recovery for humans who receive nonlethal doses of radiation in the range of 1 to 2 Gy (100 to 200 rad)? On what factors does recovery depend? If death does occur, from what does it result?

POST-TEST

The student should take this test after reading Chapter 7, finishing all accompanying textbook and workbook exercises, and completing any additional activities required by the course instructor. The student should complete the post-test with a score of 90% or higher before advancing to the next chapter. (Each of the following 20 questions or blanks is worth 5 points.) Score = _____ %

1. When biologic effects of radiation occur relatively soon after humans receive high doses of ionizing radiation, the biologic responses demonstrated are called _____.

2. What are the three separate dose-related syndromes that occur as part of the total body syndrome?

_____

_____

_____

3. Acute radiation syndrome manifests in four major response stages: _____, _____, _____, and _____ or _____.

4. When cells of the lymphatic system are damaged, the body:
   A. Increases its ability to combat infection
   B. Loses some of its ability to combat infection
   C. Manufactures large numbers of platelets to compensate for the damage
   D. Responds by repopulating mature erythrocytes in the circulating blood

5. What term is used to signify the whole-body dose of radiation that can be lethal to 50% of the exposed population within 30 days?

_____

6. Research has shown that repeated radiation injuries have a _____ effect.

7. Some local tissues experience immediate consequences from high radiation doses. Which of the following are examples of such tissues?
   1. Bone marrow
   2. Male and female reproductive organs
   3. Skin
   A. 1 and 2 only
   B. 1 and 3 only
   C. 2 and 3 only
   D. 1, 2, and 3

8. Epilation is another term for:
   A. Decrease of red blood cells
   B. Increase of white blood cells
   C. Hair loss
   D. Shedding of the outer layer of skin

9. The use of high-level fluoroscopy for extended periods of time can result in which of the following in patients?
   1. Acute radiation syndrome
   2. Repair of damaged chromosomes
   3. Radiation-induced skin injuries
   A. 1 only
   B. 2 only
   C. 3 only
   D. 1, 2, and 3

10. Define the term *nonstochastic (deterministic) somatic effects*.

_____

_____

11. What is the phase of cell division in which chromosomal damage caused by radiation exposure can be evaluated?

12. Without effective physical monitoring devices, what played an important role in the identification of radiation casualties in the first 2 days after the accident at the Chernobyl nuclear power plant?

13. The workers and firefighters at Chernobyl are examples of human beings who died as a result of _____ syndrome.

14. What is the estimated LD 50/30 for adult human beings if medical support is unavailable?

15. A cytogenetic analysis of chromosomes may be accomplished through the use of a chromosome map called a _____.

16. In females, a gonadal dose of _____ Gy (_____ rad) may delay or suppress menstruation. A single dose of _____ Gy (_____ rad) to the ovaries can result in temporary sterility, and a dose of _____ to _____ Gy (_____ to _____ rad) to the ovaries can result in permanent sterility.

17. In males, a radiation dose of _____ Gy (_____ rad) can depress the sperm population and possibly cause genetic mutations in future generations.

18. How do cells of the hematopoietic system develop?

19. The cerebrovascular form of ARS results when the central nervous and cardiovascular systems receive doses of ionizing radiation of _____ Gy (_____ rad) or higher.

20. The hematopoietic form of ARS is also called the _____.

8 Late Radiation Effects on Organ Systems

Radiation-induced damage at the cellular level may lead to measurable somatic and genetic damage in the living organism as a whole later in life. These effects are called *late effects* and refer to the long-term effects of radiation exposure. Some examples of measurable late biologic damage are cataracts, leukemia, and genetic mutations. Chapter 8 focuses on organic damage from ionizing radiation that occurs months or years later as a consequence of radiation exposure.

CHAPTER HIGHLIGHTS

- Scientists use the information from epidemiologic studies to formulate dose-response estimates to predict the risk of cancer in human populations exposed to low doses of ionizing radiation.
- Information obtained from a radiation dose-response curve can be used to predict the risk of malignancy in human populations exposed to low levels of ionizing radiation.
  - Curves that graphically demonstrate radiation dose-response relationships can be either linear or nonlinear and depict either a threshold or a nonthreshold dose.
  - A linear nonthreshold curve currently is being used for most types of cancer.
  - Risk associated with low-level radiation can be estimated with the linear-quadratic nonthreshold curve.
  - Nonstochastic (deterministic) effects of significant radiation exposure may be graphically demonstrated through the use of a linear threshold curve of radiation dose-response.
  - High-dose cellular response may be demonstrated through the use of a sigmoid threshold curve.
- Late somatic effects occur after a period of months or years after irradiation.
  - Late effects include carcinogenesis, cataractogenesis, and embryologic (birth) defects.
  - Cancer is the most important late stochastic somatic effect caused by exposure to ionizing radiation.
  - Effects directly related to dose received that occur months or years after radiation exposure are called *late nonstochastic (deterministic) somatic effects*.
  - Effects that have no threshold, occur arbitrarily, are independent of dose, and occur months or years after exposure are called *late stochastic somatic effects*.
- Risk estimates are given in terms of absolute risk or relative risk.
  - The absolute risk model predicts that a specific number of excess cancers will occur as a result of radiation exposure.
  - The relative risk model predicts that the number of excess cancers rises as the natural incidence of cancer increases with advancing age in a population.
  - Linear and linear-quadratic models are used for extrapolation of risk from high-dose to low-dose data.
- The first trimester of pregnancy is the most critical period for radiation exposure of the embryo-fetus.
  - Radiation-induced congenital abnormalities can occur 10 days to 6 weeks after conception.
  - Skeletal abnormalities most frequently occur from weeks 3 to 20.
  - Radiation exposure in the second and third trimesters can cause congenital abnormalities, functional disorders, and a predisposition to the development of childhood cancer.
- Genetic effects on ionizing radiation are biologic effects on generations yet unborn.
  - Radiation-induced abnormalities are caused by unrepaired damage to DNA within ova or sperm.
  - There is no 100% safe gonadal radiation dose; even the smallest radiation dose could cause some genetic damage.
  - Doubling dose measures the effectiveness of ionizing radiation in causing mutations; it is the radiation dose that causes the number of spontaneous mutations in a given generation to increase to two times the original number.
  - For humans, the doubling dose is estimated to have a mean value of 1.56 Sv (156 rem).

Exercise 1: Crossword Puzzle

Use the clues to complete the crossword puzzle.

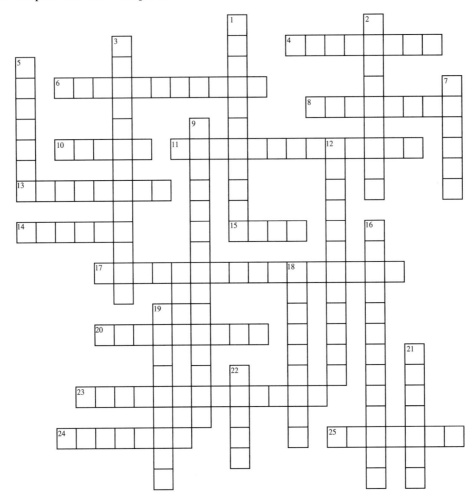

Down
1. Russian cleanup workers at Chernobyl.
2. Japanese atomic bomb survivors.
3. Status of the risk estimate for human beings of contracting cancer from low-level ionizing radiation exposure.
5. What the Navajo people of Arizona and New Mexico mined during the 1950s and 1960s for the U.S. government to meet the need for fuel for nuclear weapons and power plants.
7. Example of a stochastic somatic effect of ionizing radiation.
9. Stage when a fertilized ovum divides and forms a ball-like structure containing undifferentiated cells.
12. Relationship that means any radiation dose will produce a biologic effect.
16. Type of studies resulting from observations and statistical analysis of data, such as incidence of disease within a group of people.
18. All forms of life seem to be most vulnerable to radiation during this stage of development.
19. Not considered to be a highly effective cancer-causing agent.
21. Type of cancer that occurred in the children of the Marshall Islanders who were inadvertently subjected to high levels of fallout during an atomic bomb test in 1954.
22. Gas that decays with a half-life of 3.8 days by way of alpha particle emission.

Across

4. Axis of radiation dose-response curve that indicates biologic effects observed.
6. Mutations that occur naturally at random and without a known cause.
8. The incidence of this disease in the Japanese population after detonation of the atomic bomb was hundredfold times higher than normal because many people received high doses of radiation.
10. Project undertaken after the accident at the Chernobyl nuclear power plant to help the local population rebuild acceptable living conditions through active involvement in the reconstruction process.
11. Period of gestation in humans that corresponds to 10 days to 6 weeks postconception.
13. What agents such as elevated temperatures, ionizing radiation, viruses and chemicals that can increase the frequency of mutations in a generation of humans are called.
14. Gland that was enlarged in many infants with respiratory distress who, in the 1940s and 1950s, eventually were treated with therapeutic doses of ionizing radiation to reduce its size.
15. Nonspecialized cells derived from embryos.
17. The production or origin of cataracts.
20. Opacity of the eye lens.
23. Scaling down the risk versus dose curve from high-dose data to low doses.
24. Biologic effects of ionizing radiation on future generations.
25. Type of threshold dose-response curve that may be used to demonstrate high-dose cellular response.

Exercise 2: Matching

Match the following terms with their definitions or associated phrases.

1. _____ female Japanese atomic bomb survivors
2. _____ probabilistic effects
3. _____ fetal radiosensitivity
4. _____ radon
5. _____ linear nonthreshold dose-response curve
6. _____ relative risk model
7. _____ cancer and genetic effects
8. _____ ETHOS Project
9. _____ linear quadratic nonthreshold dose-response curve
10. _____ Thorotrast
11. _____ mutant genes
12. _____ World Health Organization
13. _____ point mutations
14. _____ skeletal
15. _____ radiobiologists
16. _____ absolute risk model
17. _____ doubling dose

A. Implies that the biologic response to ionizing radiation is directly proportional to the dose
B. A dose-response curve that is curved to some degree
C. Radioactive element with a half-life of 4.5 billion years
D. Example of stochastic effects that probably do not have a threshold
E. Another term for stochastic somatic effects
F. Predicts that a specific number of excess cancers will occur as a result of exposure to ionizing radiation
G. A 3-year research project that began in 1996 in the Republic of Belarus in the aftermath of the accident at the Chernobyl nuclear power plant
H. Reported in 1995 that nearly 700 cases of thyroid cancer among children and adolescents were linked to the Chernobyl accident
I. Radioactive contrast agent used from 1925 to 1945 that caused liver and spleen cancer in many patients after a latent period of 15 to 20 years
J. Estimates the risk associated with low-level radiation
K. Gas that emanates through tiny gaps in the rocks, creating an insidious airborne hazard to uranium miners
L. Group of people that provide strong evidence that ionizing radiation can induce breast cancer
M. Safe gonadal dose of ionizing radiation for humans
N. Predicts that the number of excess cancers will increase as the natural incidence of cancer increases with advancing age in a population
O. Genetic mutations at the molecular level
P. Mutations probably expressed in the offspring
Q. The radiation dose that causes the number of spontaneous mutations occurring in a given generation to increase to two times their original number

18. _____ linear
19. _____ dominant mutations
20. _____ recessive mutations
21. _____ nonlinear
22. _____ embryologic effects (birth effects or defects)
23. _____ uranium
24. _____ carcinogenesis
25. _____ zero

R. The production or origin of cancer
S. Decreases as gestation progresses
T. Mutations probably not expressed for several generations
U. Cannot properly govern the cell's normal chemical reactions or properly control the sequence of amino acids in the formation of specific proteins
V. People who engage in research that have a common goal to establish relationships between radiation and dose-response
W. Damage to an organism that occurs as a result of exposure to ionizing radiation during the embryonic stage of development
X. A dose-response curve that exists as a straight line
Y. Abnormalities that most frequently occur from weeks 3 to 20 of gestation in humans.

Exercise 3: Multiple Choice
Select the answer that *best* completes the following questions or statements.

1. Epidemiologic studies are of significant value to scientists who use the information from these studies to formulate dose-response estimates to predict the risk of:
   A. Cancer in human populations exposed to low doses of ionizing radiation
   B. Cataract formation in humans exposed to low doses of ionizing radiation
   C. Radiodermatitis in radiologic technologists working in the field between 1970 and 1990
   D. Radiodermatitis in radiologic technologists working in the field from 1990 to the present time

2. Which of the following measures the effectiveness of ionizing radiation in causing mutations?
   A. LD 50/30
   B. Doubling dose
   C. Relative biologic effectiveness (RBE)
   D. Dose-response curve

3. Recent studies of atomic bomb survivors tend to support the _____ risk model over the _____ risk model.
   A. Absolute, relative
   B. Relative, absolute
   C. Stochastic, nonstochastic
   D. Nonstochastic, stochastic

4. The linear dose-response model is used to establish radiation protection standards because it accurately reflects the effects of:
   A. Both high–linear energy transfer (LET) and low-LET types of radiation at higher doses
   B. Both high-LET and low-LET types of radiation at lower doses
   C. High-LET radiation at higher doses
   D. Low-LET radiation at lower doses

5. The number of excess cancers, or cancers that would *not* have occurred in a given population in question without exposure to ionizing radiation, may be predicted by which of the following?
   1. Absolute risk model
   2. Biologic risk model
   3. Relative risk model
   A. 1 and 2 only
   B. 1 and 3 only
   C. 2 and 3 only
   D. 1, 2, and 3

6. After the accident at the Chernobyl nuclear power plant in 1986, many children in Poland and some other countries were given potassium iodide in an attempt to prevent:
   A. Breast cancer
   B. Bone cancer
   C. Leukemia
   D. Thyroid cancer

7. *Most* radiation-induced genetic mutations are _____.
   A. Dominant mutations
   B. Expressed in first-generation offspring
   C. Spontaneous mutations unique to radiation
   D. Recessive mutations

8. Spontaneous mutations in human genetic material cause a wide variety of diseases including:
   1. Down syndrome
   2. Hemophilia
   3. Sickle cell anemia
   A. 1 only
   B. 2 only
   C. 3 only
   D. 1, 2, and 3

9. When exposure to ionizing radiation causes proliferation of the white blood cells, the radiation-induced disease that occurs is:
   A. Anemia
   B. Erythroleukosis
   C. Granulocytopenia
   D. Leukemia

10. Radiation can induce genetic damage by which of the following means?
    A. Interacting with somatic cells of only one parent
    B. Interacting with somatic cells of both parents
    C. Altering the essential base coding sequence of DNA
    D. None of the above; radiation cannot induce genetic damage

11. Using the doubling dose concept to measure the effectiveness of ionizing radiation at causing mutations, if 9% of the offspring in each generation are born with mutations in the absence of radiation other than background levels, administration of the doubling dose to all members of the population eventually would increase the number of mutations to:
    A. 18%
    B. 36%
    C. 72%
    D. 100%

12. Which of the following groups of individuals received radiation treatment that indicated radiation can cause breast cancer when healthy breast tissue was exposed to radiation?
    A. Female patients treated for malignant breast disease
    B. Male patients treated for malignant breast disease
    C. Patients treated for benign postpartum mastitis
    D. Radiologic technologists presently working in diagnostic imaging

13. For a recessive mutation to appear in an offspring:
    A. Both parents must have the same genetic defect
    B. Both parents must have only dominant genes
    C. Neither parent needs to have a genetic defect
    D. Only one parent must have a genetic defect

14. Based on revised atomic bomb data from Hiroshima and Nagasaki, radiation-induced leukemias and solid tumors in the survivors may be attributed predominantly to:
    A. Alpha particle exposure
    B. Beta particle exposure
    C. Gamma radiation exposure
    D. X-radiation exposure

15. After the Chernobyl nuclear power plant accident in 1986, approximately how many people worldwide received some exposure to fallout?
    A. 100,000
    B. 250,000
    C. 400,000
    D. 900,000

16. Which of the following are examples of stochastic effects?
    A. Nausea and vomiting
    B. Epilation and fatigue
    C. Diarrhea and leukopenia
    D. Cancer and genetic defects

17. During the embryonic stage of development:
    A. All life forms seem to be most vulnerable to radiation exposure
    B. Only a very small percentage of life forms seem to be vulnerable to radiation exposure
    C. A significant percentage of life forms seem to be vulnerable to radiation exposure
    D. Exposure to radiation cannot damage any life form

18. Girls who painted watch dials with radium in some factories in New Jersey in the 1920s and 1930s eventually developed which of the following conditions as a consequence of their exposure to radiation?
    1. Osteoporosis
    2. Osteogenic sarcoma
    3. Carcinomas of the epithelial lining of the nasopharynx and paranasal sinuses
    A. 1
    B. 2
    C. 3
    D. 1, 2, and 3

19. Radium decays with a half-life of 1622 years to the radioactive element:
    A. Uranium
    B. Radon
    C. Plutonium
    D. Americium

20. Mutant genes cannot properly govern the cell's normal chemical reactions or properly control the sequence of _____ in the formation of specific proteins.
    A. Amino acids
    B. Enzymes
    C. Hormones
    D. Peptic acids

21. Which of the following are mutagens?
    1. Elevated temperatures
    2. Ionizing radiation
    3. Viruses
    A. 1 and 2 only
    B. 1 and 3 only
    C. 2 and 3 only
    D. 1, 2, and 3

22. The only concrete evidence that ionizing radiation causes genetic effects comes from:
    A. Human populations exposed to low radiation doses
    B. Human populations exposed to moderate radiation doses
    C. Human populations exposed to high radiation doses
    D. Extensive experiments with fruit flies and mice at high radiation doses

23. Which of the following led to the development of the doubling dose concept?
    A. Animal studies of radiation-induced genetic effects
    B. Human studies of radiation-induced genetic effects
    C. Animal studies of radiation-induced somatic effects
    D. Human studies of radiation-induced somatic effects

24. Cataracts, leukemia, and genetic mutations are examples of:
    A. Diseases that are not caused by ionizing radiation
    B. Measurable radiation-induced biologic damage
    C. Diseases caused by nonionizing radiation
    D. Radiation-induced biologic damage that cannot be measured

25. Members of which of the following groups of radiologic technologists have the *greatest* risk of dying from breast cancer as a consequence of their occupation?
    A. Technologists who began working before 1940
    B. Technologists who began working after 1950
    C. Women employed as technologists after 1960
    D. Women employed as technologists after 2000

Exercise 4: True or False

Circle *T* if the statement is true; circle *F* if the statement is false.

1. T F Cataracts, leukemia, and genetic mutations are examples of measurable radiation-induced biologic damage.

2. T F If a threshold relationship exists between a radiation dose and a biologic response, even the smallest dose of ionizing radiation will have some biologic effect on a living organism.

3. T F The Biological Effects on Ionizing Radiation (BEIR) Committee believes that the linear-quadratic threshold curve of radiation dose-response is a more accurate reflection of stochastic somatic and genetic effects at low-dose levels from low-LET radiation.

4. T F When late effects are mutational or randomly occurring biologic somatic changes, independent of dose, they are termed *stochastic (probabilistic) somatic effects*.

5. T F Low-level doses are a consideration for patients and personnel exposed to ionizing radiation as a result of diagnostic imaging procedures.

6. T F Distinguishing radiation-induced cancer by its physical appearance is relatively easy because it looks very different from cancers caused by other agents.

7. T F Any nonlethal radiation dose received by the germ cells can cause chromosome mutations that may be transmitted to successive generations.

8. T F A genetic disorder is present in approximately 50% of all living births in the United States.

9. T F The impact of the atomic bomb dosimetry revision is a significant increase in cancer risk estimates.

10. T F Radium watch dial painters of the 1920s and 1930s provide proof of radiation cataractogenesis.

11. T F Many cases of radiation-induced skin cancer among radiation workers have been documented in recent years.

12. T F The term *linear-quadratic* means that the equation that best fits the data has terms that depend on dose (linear) and also dose squared (quadratic).

13. T F Technologists who entered the medical radiation industry in 1950 or later have demonstrated a somewhat higher risk of dying from leukemia compared with individuals who entered the workforce before 1950.

14. T F Conclusive proof exists that low-level ionizing radiation doses (i.e., those below 0.1 Sv [10 rem]) cause a significant increase in the risk of malignancy.

15. T F Reproductive cell damage that leads to impaired fertility is an example of a late deterministic somatic effect of ionizing radiation.

16. T F Irradiation of the embryo during the first 8 weeks of development with equivalent doses in excess of 200 mSv (20 rem) frequently results in death or causes congenital abnormalities.

17. T F The effect of low-level ionizing radiation on the embryo-fetus can only be estimated.

18. T F Currently, some experts theorize that all radiation exposure levels possess the potential to cause biologic damage and that radiographers must employ thoughtful radiation safety measures whenever humans are exposed to radiation during diagnostic imaging procedures.

19. T F Follow-up studies of the Japanese atomic bomb survivors of Hiroshima and Nagasaki who did not die of ARS have not demonstrated late deterministic and stochastic effects of ionizing radiation.

20. T F For humans, the doubling dose is estimated to have a mean value of 1.56 Sv (156 rem).

21. T F Information obtained from a radiation dose-response curve can be used to predict the risk of malignancy in human populations exposed to low-levels of ionizing radiation.

22. T F Currently, evidence of radiation-induced genetic effects has been observed in persons employed in diagnostic imaging and in patients undergoing radiologic examinations.

23. T F Organ atrophy is the most important late somatic effect caused by exposure to ionizing radiation.

24. T F The 1989 BEIR V Report supported use of the linear-quadratic model of radiation dose-response for leukemia only.

25. T F During the 1940s and early 1950s, to reduce an enlarged thymus gland in infants, physicians treated the babies with therapeutic doses of x-radiation (1.2 to 60 Gy [120 to 6000 rad]), resulting in a substantial dose to the nearby thyroid gland; this caused thyroid nodules and carcinomas some 20 years later.

Exercise 5: Fill in the Blank

Using the following Word Bank, fill in the blanks with the word or words that *best* complete the statements.

1.56 (156)	irradiated	reconstructing
10:1	lens	reticuloendothelial
breast	leukemia (term may be used more than once)	risk
calcium		somatic
cancer-causing		stem
cancers	linear	threshold
cellular	low	Thorotrast
damaged	malignancy	thyroid (term may be used more than once)
death	months	
first	natural	underestimate
follow-up studies	overestimate	years
genetic	radiosensitive	
iodine		

1. Radiation-induced damage at the cellular level may lead to measurable _____ and _____ damage in the living organism as a whole later in life.

2. A radiation dose-response curve is either _____ or nonlinear and depicts either a _____ dose or a nonthreshold dose.

3. In establishing radiation protection standards, the regulatory agencies have chosen to be conservative and use a model that might _____ risk but is not expected to _____ risk.

4. The incident rates at which malignancies occur as a consequence of irradiation are determined by comparing the _____ incidence of cancer occurring in a human population with the incidence of cancer occurring in an _____ population.

5. The _____ for radiation-induced cancer in radiation workers is not really measurable at _____ doses encountered in diagnostic imaging.

6. Late somatic effects are effects that appear _____ or _____ after exposure to ionizing radiation.

7. In humans, radiation-induced _____ may take 5 or more years to develop.

8. Because radium is chemically similar to _____, it was incorporated into the bone tissue of many radium watch dial painters in the early 1920s and 1930s who placed the radium-containing paint-saturated brush tip on their lips to draw the bristles of the brush to a fine point before painting the watch dial.

9. Possessing high-LET radiation, alpha particles passing through a person's lungs have a high probability of producing a great deal of _____ damage.

10. According to a recent study of 146,000 U.S. radiologic technologists, those who began working before 1940 had the greatest risk of dying of _____ cancer.

11. The mean value of the radiation doubling equivalent dose for human beings, as determined from offspring of the atomic bomb survivors of Hiroshima and Nagasaki, is _____ Sv (_____ rem).

12. From 1925 to 1945, when used as a contrast agent and administered by intravascular injection, _____, a radioactive material, emitted particles that were deposited in the patient's _____ system.

13. Radiation dose-response curves can be used to predict the risk of _____ in human populations exposed to low levels of ionizing radiation.

14. The _____ gland is adjacent to the thymus gland.

15. Numerous studies of Japanese female atomic bomb survivors have indicated a relative risk of breast cancer ranging from _____ to as high as _____.

16. Epidemiologic data on the Hiroshima atomic bomb survivors indicate that a linear relationship exists between radiation dose and radiation-induced _____.

17. Radiation actually is not a highly effective _____ agent.

18. The 1986 accident at the Chernobyl nuclear power station necessitates long-term _____ _____ to assess the magnitude and severity of late effects on the exposed population.

19. During the first 10 years after the Chernobyl disaster, the incidence of _____ cancer increased dramatically among children living in the regions of Belarus, the Ukraine, and Russia, where the heaviest radioactive _____ contamination occurred.

20. Since the Chernobyl accident, the affected population continues to work toward _____ their overall quality of life.

21. Early studies of the Chernobyl victims did not demonstrate a significant increase in the incidence of _____.

22. The _____ of the eye contains transparent fibers that transmit light.

23. Because embryonic cells begin dividing and differentiating after conception, they are extremely _____ and therefore may easily be _____ by exposure to ionizing radiation.

24. The _____ trimester of pregnancy seems to be the most crucial period with regard to irradiation of the embryo-fetus because the embryo-fetus contains a large number of _____ cells during this period of gestation.

25. During the preimplantation period (approximately 0 to 9 days after conception), the fertilized ovum divides and forms a ball-like structure containing undifferentiated cells. If this structure is irradiated with a dose in the range of 0.05 to 0.15 Gy (5 to 15 rad), embryonic _____ occurs.

Exercise 6: Labeling

Label the following illustrations and box.

A. Hypothetical radiation dose-response curves. (Hint: The terms are included in the figure legend in the textbook.)

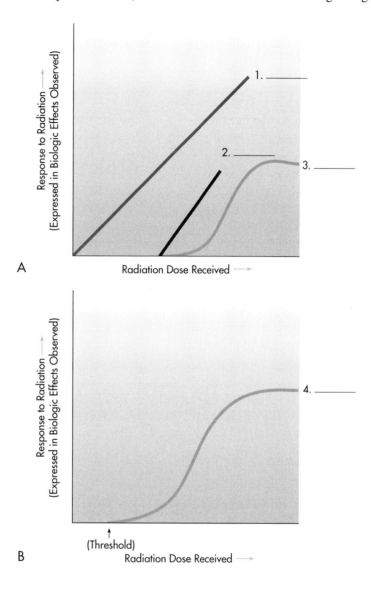

B. Hypothetical radiation dose-response curves.

Response to Radiation (Expressed in Biologic Effects)

1.
2.

Radiation Dose

C. Late somatic effects.
Late Nonstochastic Somatic Effects

1. _____

2. _____

3. _____

4. _____

5. _____

6. _____

Late Stochastic Somatic Effects

1. _____

2. _____

Exercise 7: Short Answer

Answer the following questions by providing a short answer.

1. With reference to ionizing radiation, how do threshold and nonthreshold relationships differ in terms of radiation dose and biologic response?

   _____

   _____

2. What type of experiments and data provide the foundation for a linear, threshold curve of radiation dose-response?

   _____

   _____

3. Of what do epidemiologic studies consist, and how is the risk of radiation-induced cancer determined?

4. To minimize the possibility of genetic effects in those persons engaged in the practice of medical imaging and in patients, what precautions must be taken?

5. According to members of the scientific and medical communities, what three categories of health effects related to low-level radiation exposure require further study?

6. Name three major types of late somatic effects.

7. What human evidence exists for radiation cataractogenesis?

8. What happens to fetal radiosensitivity as gestation progresses? What are the possible consequences to the developing human fetus of irradiation during the second and third trimesters of pregnancy?

9. What impact do mutagens such as ionizing radiation have on genetic mutations that occur as part of the natural order of events?

10. Name two models that researchers commonly use for extrapolation of the risk of ionizing radiation from high-dose data to low-dose data.

11. What evidence exists that ionizing radiation causes genetic effects?

12. What type of point mutations is radiation thought to cause?

13. What has led to the development of the doubling dose concept?

14. List the three stages of gestation in human beings, and identify the time period of the pregnancy to which they correspond.

15. Why were the immediate families of uranium miners extremely vulnerable to radiation-induced cancers?

Exercise 8: General Discussion or Opinion Questions

The following questions are intended to allow students to express their knowledge and understanding of the subject matter or to present a personal opinion. The questions may be used to stimulate class discussion. Because answers to these questions may vary, determination of an answer's acceptability is left to the discretion of the course instructor.

1. What is the long-range global impact of the 1986 Chernobyl nuclear power plant accident?

2. How does the radiosensitivity of the fetus during the third trimester of pregnancy compare with fetal radiosensitivity during the first trimester? What protective measures can be taken during each trimester to protect the fetus from unnecessary radiation exposure?

3. What human evidence exists that proves ionizing radiation induces cancer?

4. How is the concept of risk used to predict cancer incidence for populations exposed to ionizing radiation?

5. Using supportive information from Chapter 1 and Chapter 8, describe the ETHOS Project and explain the benefits of this project for the affected population as they work to reconstruct their overall quality of life in the aftermath of the Chernobyl nuclear power plant disaster.

POST-TEST

The student should take this test after reading Chapter 8, finishing all accompanying textbook and workbook exercises, and completing any additional activities required by the course instructor. The student should complete the post-test with a score of 90% or higher before advancing to the next chapter. (Each of the following 20 questions or blanks is worth 5 points.) Score = _____ %

1. What is the period of gestation in humans that corresponds to 10 days to 6 weeks after conception?

2. What is the most important late stochastic somatic effect of exposure to ionizing radiation?

3. When are all life forms most vulnerable to radiation exposure?

4. Using the doubling dose concept to measure the effectiveness of ionizing radiation at causing mutations, if 4% of the offspring in each generation are born with mutations in the absence of radiation other than background levels, administration of the doubling dose to all members of the population eventually would increase the number of mutations to _____%.

5. Which risk model is used to predict that a specific number of excess cancers will occur as a result of exposure to ionizing radiation?

6. Define the term *late nonstochastic (deterministic) somatic effects*.

7. Which radiation dose-response curve model implies that the biologic response to ionizing radiation is directly proportional to the dose?

8. Revised atomic bomb data for Hiroshima and Nagasaki suggest that radiation-induced leukemias and solid tumors in the survivors may be attributed predominantly to exposure to which of the following types of radiation?
   A. Alpha particles
   B. Beta particles
   C. Gamma rays
   D. Neutrons

9. Which of the following groups provide evidence for radiation carcinogenesis?
   1. Radium watch dial painters (1920s and 1930s)
   2. Early medical radiation workers (1896 to 1910)
   3. Japanese atomic bomb survivors (1945)
   A. 1 and 2 only
   B. 1 and 3 only
   C. 2 and 3 only
   D. 1, 2, and 3

10. How may risk estimates to predict cancer incidence in a population be given?

11. Where is the sigmoid, or S-shaped, (nonlinear) threshold curve of the radiation dose-response relationship generally used?

12. What incapacities are associated with mutant genes?

13. What disease occurred in the children of the Marshall Islanders who were inadvertently subjected to high levels of fallout during an atomic bomb test on March 1, 1954?

14. What does the term *linear-quadratic* mean?

15. How can ionizing radiation induce genetic damage?

16. What are mutations in genes and DNA that occur at random as a natural phenomenon?

17. According to a recent study of 146,000 U.S. radiologic technologists, those who began working before 1940 had the _____ risk of dying of breast cancer.

18. With reference to ionizing radiation, what does the term *threshold* mean?

19. The probability that a single dose of ionizing radiation of approximately _____ Gy (_____ rad) will induce the formation of cataracts is high.

20. What currently is considered the most pronounced health consequence of the radiation accident at the Chernobyl nuclear power plant?

9 Dose Limits for Exposure to Ionizing Radiation

Chapter 9 discusses occupational and nonoccupational effective dose (EfD) limits and equivalent dose (EqD) limits for tissues and organs such as the lens of the eye, skin, hands, and feet. To minimize the risk of harmful biologic effects, exposure of the general public, patients, and radiation workers to ionizing radiation must be limited through adherence to established dose limits. The effective dose limiting system, a set of numeric dose limits that are based on calculations of the various risks of cancer and genetic effects caused by exposure to radiation, have been established for this purpose. This chapter also covers organizations responsible for radiation protection standards and U.S. regulatory agencies. The current radiation protection philosophy is discussed, and goals and objectives for radiation protection are identified. Other topics include the concept of as low as reasonably achievable (ALARA), the responsibilities of a radiation safety officer, the risk of radiation-induced malignancy, action limits, and the theory of radiation hormesis.

CHAPTER HIGHLIGHTS

- Effective dose limiting system:
  - Adherence to occupational and nonoccupational effective dose limits helps prevent harmful biologic effects of radiation exposure.
  - The concept of radiation exposure and associated risk of radiation-induced malignancy is the basis of the effective dose limiting system.
  - The sum of both external and internal whole-body exposures is considered during establishment of the effective dose limit.
  - Accounting for tissue weighting factors is important because various tissues and organs do not have the same degree of sensitivity.
  - Different biologic threats posed by different types of ionizing radiation must be taken into consideration even when the absorbed dose is the same.
- Radiation hormesis is the hypothesis that a positive effect exists for certain populations that are continuously exposed to moderate levels of radiation.
- Major organizations involved in regulating radiation exposure include:
  - UNSCEAR and NAS/NRC-BEIR supply information to the ICRP.
  - The ICRP makes recommendations on occupational and public dose limits.
  - The NCRP reviews the ICRP recommendations and implements them into U.S. radiation protection policy.
  - The NRC is the watchdog of the nuclear energy industry; it controls the manufacture and use of radioactive substances.
  - The EPA develops and enforces regulations pertaining to the control of environmental radiation.
  - The FDA regulates the design and manufacture of products used in the radiation industry.
  - OSHA monitors the workplace and regulates occupational exposure to radiation.
- Individual health care facilities establish an RSC and designate an RSO.
  - The RSO is responsible for developing a radiation safety program for the health care facility; he or she maintains personnel radiation-monitoring records and provides counseling in radiation safety.
- The ALARA concept (optimization) states that radiation exposure should be kept "as low as reasonably achievable."
- Serious radiation-induced responses may be classified as having either nonstochastic or stochastic effects.
  - Nonstochastic effects are those biologic somatic effects of ionizing radiation that exhibit a threshold dose below which the effect does not normally occur and above which the severity of the biologic damage increases as the dose increases.
  - Stochastic effects are nonthreshold, randomly occurring biologic somatic changes in which the chance of occurrence of the effect rather than the severity of the effect is proportional to the dose of ionizing radiation.
- Effective dose limit:
  - The NCRP has established an annual occupational effective dose limit of 50 mSv (5 rem) and a guideline that lifetime effective dose not exceed 10 times the occupationally exposed person's age in years.
  - Collective effective dose is used in the description of population or group exposure to low doses of different sources of ionizing radiation.
  - Internal action limits are established by health care facilities to trigger an investigation to uncover the reasons for any unusual high exposures received by individual staff members.

Exercise 1: Crossword Puzzle

Use the clues to complete the crossword puzzle.

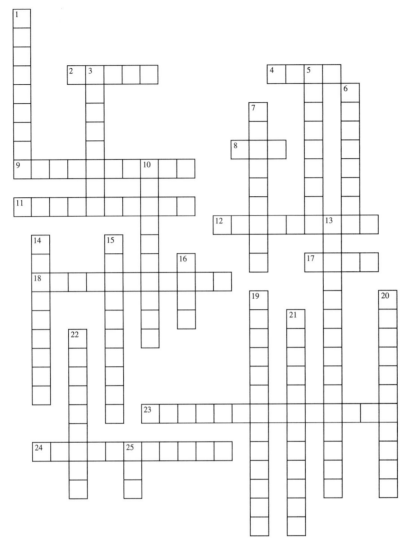

Down

1. Loss of hair.
3. The type of effective dose that must be limited to a radiation worker's age in years times 10 mSv (years × 1 rem).
5. City in Japan on which an atomic bomb was dropped.
6. Levels of ionizing radiation formerly considered acceptable by the ICRP have been revised in this direction.
7. Where OSHA regulates training programs.
10. Type of consequence of radiation for populations continuously exposed to moderately high levels of radiation that suggest a potential radiation hormesis effect.
13. What government organizations use from NCRP as the scientific basis for their radiation protection activities.
14. States in the United States that can enter into contract with the Nuclear Regulatory Commission to assume the responsibility for enforcing radiation protection regulations through their respective health departments.
15. Effects that occur randomly in nature and whose severity is not dose dependent.
16. What the benefit obtained from any diagnostic imaging procedure must always be weighed against.
19. Type of act that establishes limits on radiation exposure.
20. Type of authority an RSO must have in a health care facility to stop unsafe operations.
21. Types of states in which both the state and the NRC enforce radiation protection regulations by sending agents to health care facilities.
22. What the risk of cancer induction from low absorbed doses of ionizing radiation can only be at the present time.
25. Agency established in 1970 to bring several agencies under one organization that would be responsible for protecting the health of human beings and for safeguarding the natural environment.

Across

2. As low as reasonably achievable.
4. Functions as a monitoring agency in places of employment predominantly in industry.
8. Formerly known as the Atomic Energy Commission (AEC).
9. What deterministic effects such as mental retardation are expected to be, if the equivalent dose remains below the established limit.
11. Regarding the protection of radiation workers, and the population as a whole, this is what effective dose limits have been established to serve as.
12. What the NRC writes that are presented as rules and regulations.
17. Determines the way ICRP recommendations are incorporated into United States radiation protection criteria.
18. The NRC licenses users of this type of material.
23. Implementation of an effective radiation safety program in a health care facility begins with this department.
24. Irradiation of reproductive cells before conception.

Exercise 2: Matching

Match the following terms with their definitions or associated phrases.

1. _____ NCRP Report No. 116 *(Limitation of Exposure to Ionizing Radiation)*
2. _____ EfD limiting system
3. _____ EfD
4. _____ ICRP
5. _____ RSO
6. _____ UNSCEAR
7. _____ negligible individual dose (NID)
8. _____ annual occupational EfD limit
9. _____ ALARA concept
10. _____ ColEfD
11. _____ § 10 CFR 35.50 and § 10 CFR 35.900 of the *Code of Federal Regulations*
12. _____ Annals of ICRP
13. _____ action limits
14. _____ Radiation Control for Health and Safety Act of 1968 (Public Law 90-602)

A. Cancerous neoplasms caused by exposure to ionizing radiation
B. Optimization for radiation protection.
C. Training and experience required for an RSO.
D. Strictly an equipment performance standard.
E. Agency that has the power to enforce radiation protection standards.
F. Indicates the ratio of the risk of stochastic effects attributed to irradiation of a given organ or tissue to the total risk when the whole body is uniformly irradiated.
G. Leading international organization responsible for providing clear, consistent radiation guidance through its recommendations on occupational and public dose limits.
H. Lifetime EfD.
I. Describes the level of radiation exposure of a population or group from low doses of different sources of ionizing radiation.
J. Evaluates human and environmental exposure to ionizing radiation from a variety of sources, including radioactive materials, radiation-producing machines, and radiation accidents.
K. Responsible for regulations concerning employees' right to know about hazards that may be present in the workplace.
L. Federal legislation requiring the establishment of minimal standards for the accreditation of educational programs for personnel who perform radiologic procedures and the certification of such individuals.
M. Established by health care facilities to trigger an investigation to uncover the reasons for any unusual high exposure received by individual staff members.
N. Set of numeric dose limits that are based on calculations of the various risks of cancer and genetic effects to tissues or organs exposed to radiation.

15. _____ OSHA

16. _____ BEIR reports

17. _____ FDA

18. _____ EfD limit

19. _____ NRC

20. _____ cumulative effective dose (CumEfD) limit

21. _____ EqD limit

22. _____ tissue weighting factor (W_T)

23. _____ radiation-induced malignancy

24. _____ Consumer-Patient Radiation Health and Safety Act (Title IX of Public Law 97-35).

25. _____ Code of standards for diagnostic x-ray equipment

O. Conducts an ongoing products radiation control program, regulating the design and manufacture of electronic products, including diagnostic x-ray equipment.

P. An upper boundary limit for radiation workers for yearly whole-body exposure (excluding personal medical and natural background exposure) of 50 mSv (5 rem).

Q. An annual EfD that provides a low-exposure cutoff level so that regulatory agencies may dismiss a level of individual risk as negligible.

R. Normally a medical physicist, health physicist, radiologist, or other individual qualified through adequate training and experience who is designated by a health care facility and approved by the NRC and the state to ensure that a facility follows internationally accepted guidelines for radiation protection.

S. Scientific journals published by the ICRP.

T. A quantity that is used for radiation protection purposes to provide a measure of the overall risk of exposure to ionizing radiation. This quantity takes into account the dose of all types of ionizing radiation to irradiated organs or tissues in the human body. By including a specific weighting factor for each irradiated body part, EfD takes into account the chance of each part for developing a radiation-induced cancer (or, in the case of the reproductive organs, the risk for genetic damage).

U. Publications that list studies of biologic effects and associated risk of groups of people who were either routinely or accidentally exposed to ionizing radiation.

V. EfD recommended as an upper boundary dose of ionizing radiation that results in a negligible risk of bodily injury or genetic damage.

W. Applies to complete x-ray systems and major components manufactured after August 1, 1974.

X. Provides the most recent guidance on radiation protection.

Y. A radiation quantity used for radiation protection purposes when a person receives exposure from various types of ionizing radiation. This quantity attempts to numerically specify the differences in biologic harm that are produced by different types of radiation. This quantity is the product of the average absorbed dose in a tissue or organ in the human body and the associated radiation weighting factor chosen for the type of radiation in question.

Exercise 3: Multiple Choice

Select the answer that *best* completes the following questions or statements.

1. Why have scientists developed occupational and nonoccupational effective dose limits?
   A. To eliminate all harmful effects of low-level ionizing radiation exposure
   B. To minimize the risk of harmful biologic effects to the general public, patients, and radiation workers
   C. To promote radiation hormesis
   D. To be comparable to the risk occurring in both nonsafe and safe industries

2. Which of the following concerns the upper boundary dose of ionizing radiation that results in a *negligible risk* of bodily injury or genetic damage?
   A. Skin erythema dose
   B. Dose limits
   C. ColEfD
   D. EfD limit

3. Fundamental radiation protection standards governing occupational radiation exposure may be found in which of the following documents?
   A. 5 CFR 10
   B. 10 CFR 20
   C. *The ALARA Manual*
   D. Public Law 90-602

4. Which of the following groups are radiation protection standards organizations?
   1. ICRP
   2. NCRP
   3. UNSCEAR
   A. 1 and 2 only
   B. 1 and 3 only
   C. 2 and 3 only
   D. 1, 2, and 3

5. The NCRP recommends that radiation exposure be kept at which of the following levels?
   A. As low as reasonably achievable
   B. At threshold levels
   C. Slightly above upper boundary levels
   D. At 0.01 mSv/yr

6. Which of the following concepts is behind the establishment of the effective dose limiting system?
   A. Negligible risk
   B. Organ and tissue radiosensitivity
   C. Radiation hormesis
   D. Radiation exposure and associated risk of possible radiation-induced malignancy

7. The term *mutagenesis* refers to which of the following?
   A. Birth defects from irradiation of reproductive cells before conception
   B. Birth defects from irradiation of the unborn child in utero
   C. Cancer caused by ionizing radiation exposure
   D. Somatic effects of ionizing radiation caused by low-level exposure

8. Somatic effects of ionizing radiation that exhibit a threshold dose *below* which the effect does not normally occur and *above* which the severity of the biologic damage *increases* as the dose *increases* are classified as which of the following?
   A. Deterministic effects
   B. Epidemiologic effects
   C. Probabilistic effects
   D. Stochastic effects

9. Congress passed the Radiation Control for Health and Safety Act (Public Law 90-602) in 1968 to protect the public from the hazards of unnecessary radiation exposure resulting from which of the following?
   A. Diagnostic x-ray equipment only
   B. Therapeutic x-ray equipment only
   C. Electronic products, excluding diagnostic x-ray equipment
   D. Electronic products, including diagnostic x-ray equipment

10. Which of the following are classified as *late* deterministic somatic effects?
    1. Cataract formation
    2. Organ atrophy
    3. Radiation-induced malignancy
    A. 1 and 2 only
    B. 1 and 3 only
    C. 2 and 3 only
    D. 1, 2, and 3

11. What term is used for a *beneficial* effect of radiation in populations continuously exposed to low levels of radiation above background?
    A. Nonoccupational EqD effect
    B. Radiation negligible risk level effect
    C. Radiation hormesis effect
    D. Radiation benevolent effect

12. In addition to the annual occupational effective dose limit established for radiation workers, the NCRP recommends a lifetime effective dose limit, which is found by multiplying a person's age in years by which of the following?
    A. 1 mSv (0.1 rem)
    B. 10 mSv (1 rem)
    C. 100 mSv (10 rem)
    D. 1000 mSv (100 rem)

13. For members of the general public not occupationally exposed, the NCRP recommends an annual effective dose limit of _____ for continuous (or frequent) exposures from artificial sources of ionizing radiation other than medical irradiation and natural background and a limit of _____ annually for infrequent exposures.
    A. 1 mSv (0.1 rem), 5 mSv (0.5 rem)
    B. 3 mSv (0.3 rem), 8 mSv (0.8 rem)
    C. 10 mSv (1 rem), 20 mSv (2 rem)
    D. 50 mSv (5 rem), 75 mSv (7.5 rem)

14. Which of the following is the unit of choice for expressing the collective effective dose?
    A. Group-gray (group-rad)
    B. Person-coulomb per kilogram (person-roentgen)
    C. Person-sievert (man-rem)
    D. Group-coulomb (group-roentgen)

15. A set of numeric dose limits that are based on calculations of the various risks of cancer and genetic effects to tissues or organs exposed to radiation defines
    A. ALARA concept
    B. Effective dose limiting system
    C. Investigational levels
    D. Risk protocol

16. Previously, the NRC was known as the:
    A. AEC
    B. EPA
    C. FDA
    D. OSHA

17. The Radiation Effects Research Foundation is a group run by the government of:
    A. The United States to study the effects of low-level ionizing radiation on populations
    B. Germany to study the effects of ionizing radiation on the population
    C. Japan, primarily to study the atomic bomb survivors of Hiroshima and Nagasaki
    D. England to study the development of childhood cancer in children exposed in utero to ionizing radiation

18. Person-sievert (man-rem) may be used to express:
    A. Annual occupational EfD for radiation workers
    B. ColEfD
    C. CumEfD
    D. EqD

19. Which agency is responsible for regulations regarding employees' right to know about hazards that may be present in the workplace?
    A. NRC
    B. All NRC agreement states
    C. EPA
    D. OSHA

20. The conclusions of BEIR Report No. 5 about the adverse health effects of low levels of ionizing radiation are based on extrapolations from radiation equivalent dose greater than:
    A. 1 mSv (0.1 rem)
    B. 0.1 Sv (10 rem)
    C. 50 mSv (5 rem)
    D. 0.5 Sv (50 rem)

21. Because the tissue weighting factors (W_T) used to calculate effective dose are so small for some organs, an organ associated with a low weighting factor may receive an unreasonably large dose even though the effective dose remains within the allowable total limit. Therefore special limits are set for the crystalline lens of the eye and localized areas of the skin, hands, and feet to prevent:
    1. Nonstochastic effects
    2. Stochastic effects
    3. Probabilistic effects
    A. 1 only
    B. 2 only
    C. 3 only
    D. 1, 2, and 3

22. Late deterministic somatic effects (e.g., cataract formation) have a high probability of occurring when entrance radiation doses exceed:
    A. 0.05 Gy (5 rad)
    B. 0.5 Gy (50 rad)
    C. 1 Gy (100 rad)
    D. 2 Gy (200 rad)

23. Established organ or tissue weighting factors for calculating the effective dose include a "remainder" that takes into account additional tissues and organs, some of which are the:
    1. Brain
    2. Small intestine and large intestine
    3. Uterus
    A. 1 and 2 only
    B. 1 and 3 only
    C. 2 and 3 only
    D. 1, 2, and 3

24. In International System (SI) units, the cumulative effective dose limit for the whole body of an occupationally exposed person who is 26 years old is:
    A. 26 mSv
    B. 260 mSv
    C. 2600 mSv
    D. 26,000 mSv

25. In traditional system units, the cumulative effective dose limit for the whole body of a 26-year-old occupationally exposed individual is:
    A. 2.6 rem
    B. 26 rem
    C. 260 rem
    D. 2600 rem

Exercise 4: True or False

Circle *T* if the statement is true; circle *F* if the statement is false.

1. T F The ICRP functions as an enforcement agency for radiation protection purposes.

2. T F Future radiation protection standards are expected to continue to be based on risk.

3. T F The Radiation Effects Research Foundation is a group run by the government of Japan primarily for the purpose of studying the atomic bomb survivors.

4. T F The NRC regulates and inspects x-ray imaging facilities.

5. T F In 1991 the ICRP recommended the reduction of the annual effective dose limit for occupationally exposed persons from 50 mSv (5 rem) to 20 mSv (2 rem) as a result of new information obtained from the Japanese atomic bomb survivors; this information indicated that the radiation damage done by the atomic bomb detonations was approximately three to four times greater (more damaging) that previously believed.

6. T F Health care facilities that provide imaging services do not need to have an effective radiation safety program.

7. T F Effective dose limits may be expressed for whole-body exposure, partial-body exposure, and exposure of individual organs.

8. T F Radiation risks are derived from the complete injury caused by radiation exposure.

9. T F The Center for Devices and Radiological Health (CDRH) is responsible for credentialing radiographers.

10. T F Late deterministic somatic effects may occur months or years after high-level radiation exposure.

11. T F The ICRP is considered the international authority on the safe use of sources of ionizing radiation.

12. T F The NRC publishes rules and regulations in Title X of the *Code of Federal Regulations*.

13. T F The FDA facilitates the development and enforcement of regulations pertaining to the control of radiation in the environment.

14. T F For high–dose-rate fluoroscopic procedures, entrance exposure rates as great as 20 R/min are not uncommon.

15. T F Health care facilities, such as hospitals, set their own internal action limits.

16. T F A stochastic event is an all-or-none response, meaning that ionizing radiation could cause a disease process (e.g., cancer) in the general population.

17. T F The embryo-fetus is particularly insensitive to radiation exposure.

18. T F Effective dose limits include radiation exposure from natural background radiation and exposure acquired when a worker undergoes medical imaging procedures.

19. T F To reduce exposure of pregnant female radiation workers and to control exposure of the unborn during potentially sensitive periods of gestation, the NCRP now recommends a monthly equivalent dose limit to the embryo-fetus not to exceed 0.5 mSv (0.05 rem) and a limit during the entire pregnancy not to exceed 5.0 mSv (0.50 rem) after declaration of pregnancy.

20. T F In a health care facility, the RSO is meant to be a passive participant, along with the imaging department manager, in an ongoing program that prevents personnel from receiving anywhere near the maximum allowed exposures.

21. T F Lifetime survival data appear to indicate that Japanese atomic bomb survivors with moderate radiation exposure of 5 to 50 mSv (0.5 to 5 rem), the equivalent of 1.5 to 15 years of natural radiation, have a reduced cancer death rate compared with a normally exposed control population.

22. T F Employers are not required by law to evaluate their workplace for hazardous agents or to provide training and written information to their employees.

23. T F The CDRH falls under the jurisdiction of the FDA.

24. T F Radiation hormesis is the hypothesis that a positive effect exists for certain populations that are continuously exposed to moderate levels of radiation.

25. T F All imaging personnel should be familiar with NCRP recommendations.

Exercise 5: Fill in the Blank

Using the following Word Bank, fill in the blanks with the word or words that best complete the statements.

0.4 (40)	genetic	previous
1 (0.1)	greater	radiation safety
8	internal	radioactive
10	linear	radon
15	linear quadratic	random
50 (5)	mutations	risk (term may be used
biologic	new	more than once)
cancer	nongovernmental	same
dose limits (term may be	nonoccupationally	stochastic
used more than once)	nonprofit	whole body
existing	optimization	
external		

1. Because medical imaging professionals share the responsibility for patient safety from radiation exposure and also are subject to such exposure in the performance of their duties, they must be familiar with _____, _____, and _____ guidelines.

2. Since its inception in 1928, the ICRP has been the leading international organization responsible for providing clear and consistent radiation protection guidance through its recommendations on occupational and public _____ _____.

3. In the United States the NCRP is a _____, _____ private corporation.

4. NAS/NRC-BEIR is an advisory group that reviews studies of _____ effects of ionizing radiation and _____ assessment.

5. The EPA has the authority for determining the action level for _____.

6. The NRC licenses users of _____ materials.

7. The NRC mandates that a _____ _____ committee be established for a facility to assist in the development of a radiation safety program.

8. Separate _____ _____ are set for occupationally exposed individuals and for the general public.

9. ALARA may also be referred to as _____.

10. Cancer and genetic alterations are examples of _____ effects.

11. The limit for any education and training exposures of individuals under the age of 18 is an effective dose of _____ mSv (_____ rem) annually.

12. The ALARA concept presents an extremely conservative model with respect to the relationship between ionizing radiation and potential _____.

13. Because stochastic effects are _____, determining which members of an exposed population will develop cancer is not possible before the radiation dose is received.

14. When ionizing radiation damages reproductive cells, _____ may develop that could bring an injurious consequence in subsequent generations.

15. Currently, the risk of cancer induction from low absorbed doses of ionizing radiation can only be estimated by extrapolating (scaling down) from high-dose data, using either a _____ or _____ _____ model.

16. Revised concepts of radiation exposure and _____ have brought about recent changes in NCRP recommendations for limits on exposure to ionizing radiation.

17. The lifetime fatal risk in hazardous occupations such as logging and deep-sea fishing is many times _____ than the occupational risk associated with radiation exposure.

18. Epidemiologic studies of atomic bomb survivors exposed in utero have provided conclusive evidence of a dose-dependent increase in the incidence of severe mental retardation for fetal doses greater than approximately _____ Sv (_____ rem).

19. Referring to statement 18 above, the greatest risk for radiation-induced mental retardation was found to occur when the embryo-fetus was exposed _____ to _____ weeks after conception.

20. The effective dose limiting system is an attempt to equate the various risks of _____ and _____ effects to the tissues or organs that were exposed to radiation.

21. The cumulative effective dose limit pertains to the _____ _____.

22. In addition to limits for occupationally exposed individuals, the NCRP also sets limits for _____ exposed individuals who are not undergoing medical examinations. An example of such persons would be a spouse, parent, or guardian accompanying a patient to the radiology department.

23. For education and training purposes, the same dose limits should apply to students of radiography in general and to individuals under 18 years of age. The dose limit is the _____ for kindergarten through twelfth-grade students attending science demonstrations involving ionizing radiation as it is for radiologic technologists under the age of 18.

24. The sum of both _____ and _____ whole-body exposures is considered when an effective dose limit is being established.

25. The NCRP has established an annual occupational effective dose limit of _____ mSv (_____ rem) and a lifetime effective dose that does not exceed _____ times the occupationally exposed person's age in years.

Exercise 6: Labeling
Label the following tables.

A. Summary of radiation protection standards organizations.

Organization	Function
1. _____	Evaluates information on biologic effects of radiation and provides radiation protection guidance through general recommendations on occupational and public dose limits
2. _____	Reviews regulations formulated by the ICRP and decides ways to include those recommendations in U.S. radiation protection criteria
3. _____	Evaluates human and environmental ionizing radiation exposure and derives radiation risk assessments from epidemiologic data and research conclusions; provides information to organizations such as the ICRP for evaluation
4. _____	Reviews studies of biologic effects of ionizing radiation and risk assessment and provides the information to organizations such as the ICRP for evaluation

B. Summary of U.S. regulatory agencies.

Agency	Function
1. _____	Oversees the nuclear energy industry; enforces radiation protection standards; publishes its rules and regulations in Title 10 of the U.S. Code of Federal Regulations; enters into written agreements with state governments, permitting the state to license and regulate the use of radioisotopes and certain other material within that state
2. _____	Enforces radiation protection regulations through their respective health departments
3. _____	Facilitates the development and enforcement of regulations pertaining to the control of radiation in the environment
4. _____	Conducts an ongoing product radiation control program, regulating the design and manufacture of electronic products, including x-ray equipment
5. _____	Functions as a monitoring agency in places of employment, predominantly in industry

C. Summary of National Council on Radiation Protection and Measurements (NCRP) Recommendations*† (NCRP Report No. 116).

A. Occupational exposures‡		
1. Effective dose limits		
a. Annual	1. __ mSv	(__ rem)
b. Cumulative	2. __ mSv × age	__ rem × age
2. Equivalent dose annual limits for tissues and organs		
a. Lens of eye	3. __ mSv	(__ rem)
b. Localized areas of the skin, hands, and feet	4. __ mSv	(__ rem)
B. Guidance for emergency occupational exposure‡ (see Section 14, NCRP Report No. 116)		
C. Public exposures (annual)		
1. Effective dose limit, continuous or frequent exposure‡	5. __ mSv	(__ rem)
2. Effective dose limit, infrequent exposure‡	6. __ mSv	(__ rem)
3. Equivalent dose limits for tissues and organs‡		
a. Lens of eye	7. __ mSv	(__ rem)
b. Localized areas of the skin, hands, and feet	8. __ mSv	(__ rem)
4. Remedial action for natural sources		
a. Effective dose (excluding radon)	9. >__ mSv	(>__ rem)
b. Exposure to radon and its decay products§	10. >__ J/(sm^{-3})‖	(__ WLM)
D. Education and training exposures (annual)‡		
1. Effective dose limit	11. __ mSv	(__ rem)
2. Equivalent dose limit for tissues and organs		
a. Lens of eye	12. __ mSv	(__ rem)
b. Localized areas of the skin, hands, and feet	13. __ mSv	(__ rem)
E. Embryo-fetus exposures‡		
1. Equivalent dose limit		
a. Monthly	14. __ mSv	(__ rem)
b. Entire gestation	15. __ mSv	(__ rem)
F. Negligible individual dose (annual)‡	16. __ mSv	(__ rem)

*Excluding medical exposures.
†See Tables 4.2 and 5.1 in NCRP Report No. 116 for recommendations on radiation weighting factors and tissue weighting factors, respectively.
‡Sum of external and internal exposures, excluding doses from natural sources.
§WLM stands for *working level month* and refers to a cumulative exposure for a working month (170 hours). As applied to radon and its daughter products, 1 WLM represents the cumulative exposure experienced in a 170-hour period resulting from a radon concentration of 100 pCi/L. The occupational limit for miners is 4 WLM per year, which results in a dose equivalent of approximately 0.15 Sv (15 rem) per year.
‖A measure of the rate of release of energy (joules per second) by radon and its decay products per unit volume of air (cubic meters).

Exercise 7: Short Answer

Answer the following questions by providing a short answer.

1. What have scientists developed to limit radiation exposure of the general public, patients, and radiation workers?

_____

_____

2. Why must medical imaging professionals be familiar with previous, existing, and new radiation safety guidelines?

_____

_____

3. Name four major organizations responsible for evaluating the relationship between radiation equivalent dose and induced biologic effects.

4. Name five U.S. regulatory agencies responsible for enforcing radiation protection standards to safeguard the general public, patients, and occupationally exposed personnel.

5. Why should a health care facility have a radiation safety committee?

6. What are the training and experience requirements for a RSO?

7. How do health care facilities define ALARA?

8. List two specific radiation protection objectives.

9. How is the occupational risk associated with radiation exposure equated?

10. Why haven't all U.S. states complied with the Consumer-Patient Radiation Health and Safety Act of 1981?

11. Give an example of a mutation that could cause radiation damage to reproductive cells in subsequent generations.

12. Give two inclusive categories that encompass the radiation-induced responses of serious concern in radiation protection programs.

13. What is the purpose of the Consumer-Patient Radiation Health and Safety Act of 1981?

14. The EPA was established for what purpose?

15. Define the term *exposure linearity*.

Exercise 8: General Discussion or Opinion Questions

The following questions are intended to allow students to express their knowledge and understanding of the subject matter or to present a personal opinion. The questions may be used to stimulate class discussion. Because answers to questions may vary, determination of the answer's acceptability is left to the discretion of the course instructor.

1. How does current radiation protection philosophy affect patient and personnel radiation exposure?

2. Using concept of radiation hormesis and data from any available studies, explain how radiation could possibly have a beneficial consequence for a group or population.

3. What are some of the important provisions of the code of standards for diagnostic x-ray equipment that went into effect on August 1, 1974? How do these standards improve radiation safety?

4. What does the process of assessing the risk of cancer induction from high and low doses of ionizing radiation involve?

5. Since 2008, what changes have been made in the Nuclear Regulatory Commission's scope of responsibility?

Exercise 9: Calculation Problems

Solve the following problems.

A radiation worker's lifetime effective dose must be limited to his or her age in years times 10 mSv (years × 1 rem). This is the cumulative effective limit, which pertains to the whole body. Adherence to the limit ensures that the lifetime risk for these workers remains acceptable. The following problems demonstrate the application of the cumulative effective dose limit. In the problems, equivalent dose represents the cumulative effective dose.

1. Using the SI system, determine the cumulative effective dose limit (in mSv) for the whole body of an occupationally exposed person who is 54 years old.

2. Using the traditional system, determine the cumulative effective dose limit (in rem) for the whole body of an occupationally exposed person who is 54 years old.

3. Using the SI system, determine the cumulative effective dose limit (in mSv) for the whole body of an occupationally exposed person who is 46 years old.

4. Using the traditional system, determine the cumulative effective dose limit (in rem) for the whole body of an occupationally exposed person who is 46 years old.

5. Using the SI system, determine the cumulative effective dose limit (in mSv) for the whole body of an occupationally exposed person who is 33 years old.

6. Using the traditional system, determine the cumulative effective dose limit (in rem) for the whole body of an occupationally exposed person who is 33 years old.

7. Using the SI system, determine the cumulative effective dose limit (in mSv) for the whole body of an occupationally exposed person who is 25 years old.

8. Using the traditional system, determine the cumulative effective dose limit (in rem) for the whole body of an occupationally exposed person who is 25 years old.

9. Using the SI system, determine the cumulative effective dose limit (in mSv) for the whole body of an occupationally exposed person who is 18 years old.

10. Using the traditional system, determine the cumulative effective dose limit (in rem) for the whole body of an occupationally exposed person who is 18 years old.

POST-TEST

The student should take this test after reading Chapter 9, finishing all accompanying textbook and workbook exercises, and completing any additional activities required by the course instructor. The student should complete the post-test with a score of 90% or higher before advancing to the next chapter. (Each of the following 20 questions or blanks is worth 5 points.) Score = _____ %

1. Define *risk* as it relates to the radiation sciences.

2. The NRC is a federal agency that has the authority to control the possession, use, and production of atomic energy in the interest of _____ _____.

3. What U.S. agency functions as a monitoring agency in places of employment, predominantly in industry?

4. In a health care facility, who is responsible for developing an appropriate radiation safety program to ensure that all people are adequately protected from radiation?

5. Using the SI system, determine the cumulative effective dose limit (in mSv) for the whole body of an occupationally exposed person who is 39 years old.

6. Using the traditional system, determine the cumulative effective dose limit (in rem) for the whole body of an occupationally exposed person who is 39 years old.

7. What system is the current method for assessing radiation exposure and the associated risk of biologic damage to radiation workers and the general public?

8. ALARA is the acronym for what term?

9. Biologic somatic effects of ionizing radiation that can be directly related to the dose received are called:
    1. Deterministic effects
    2. Stochastic effects
    3. Nonstochastic effects
   A. 1 and 2 only
   B. 1 and 3 only
   C. 2 and 3 only
   D. 1, 2, and 3

10. Examples of stochastic effects include
    1. Acute radiation syndrome
    2. Cancer
    3. Genetic alterations
    A. 1 and 2 only
    B. 1 and 3 only
    C. 2 and 3 only
    D. 1, 2, and 3

11. Currently the risk of cancer induction from low absorbed doses of ionizing radiation can only be _____ by extrapolating (scaling down) from high-dose data using either a linear or a linear quadratic model.

12. The current radiation protection philosophy is based on the assumption that a _____ _____ relationship exists between radiation dose and biologic response.

13. With what may the occupational risk associated with radiation exposure be equated?

14. What essential concept underlies radiation protection?

15. What dose limit does the NCRP recommend as an equivalent dose limit for the embryo-fetus during the entire period of gestation?

16. The annual occupational effective dose that applies to radiographers during routine operations is _____.

17. Why is accounting for tissue weighting factors important?

18. Adherence to occupational and nonoccupational _____ dose limits helps prevent harmful biologic effects of radiation exposure.

19. What is radiation hormesis?

20. Why are internal action limits established by health care facilities?

10 Equipment Design for Radiation Protection

Chapter 10 covers state-of-the-art diagnostic radiographic and fluoroscopic equipment that has been designed with many devices that radiologists and imaging personnel can use to optimize the quality of the image and also reduce radiation exposure for patients undergoing various imaging procedures. Although many safety features have been built into x-ray–producing machines by their manufacturers to ensure radiation safety, some features have also been included to meet federal regulations. In addition to imaging equipment, many accessories are also available to lower radiation dose for the patient. This chapter provides an overview of imaging equipment components and accessories that imaging professionals can use to minimize radiation exposure to patients during diagnostic x-ray procedures.

CHAPTER HIGHLIGHTS

- A diagnostic-type protective tube housing protects the patient and imaging personnel from off-focus, or leakage, radiation by restricting the emission of x-rays to the area of the useful, or primary, beam.
  - Leakage radiation from the tube housing measured at 1 m (3.3 feet) from the x-ray source must not exceed 100 mR/h (2.58×10^{-5} C/kg)/h when the tube is operated at its highest voltage at the highest current that allows continuous operation.
- The control panel must be located behind a suitable protective barrier that has a radiation-absorbent window that permits observation of the patient during any procedure.
  - This panel must "indicate the conditions of exposure and must positively indicate when the x-ray tube is energized."*
- The radiographic examination tabletop must be of the same thickness and be as radiolucent as possible so that it will absorb only a minimal amount of radiation, thereby reducing the patient's radiation dose.
  - The tabletop is frequently made of a carbon fiber material.
- Radiographic equipment must have a source-to–image receptor distance (SID) indicator.
- X-ray beam limitation devices must be used to confine the useful beam before it enters the anatomic area of clinical interest.
  - The light-localizing variable-aperture rectangular collimator, aperture diaphragms, cones, and cylinders are the beam limitation devices used.
  - The patient's skin surface should always be at least 15 cm below the collimator so that exposure to the epidermis is minimized.
  - Good coincidence between the x-ray beam and the light-localizing beam of the collimator is necessary; both alignment and width dimensions of the two beams must correspond to within 2% of the SID.
  - According to most state regulatory standards presently in effect, 2% of the SID is required with PBL devices. Some states may require 3% of the SID with PBL devices.
- Exposure to the patient's skin may be reduced through proper filtration of the radiographic beam.
  - Inherent filtration amounting to 0.5 mm aluminum equivalent is required.
  - Together, the inherent and added filtration comprise the total filtration. Stationary x-ray units operating above 70 kVp are required to have a total filtration of 2.5 mm aluminum equivalent.
  - The HVL of the beam is measured to determine whether an x-ray beam is adequately filtered.
- Compensating filters are used in radiography to provide uniform imaging of body parts when considerable variation in thickness or tissue composition exists.
- Diagnostic x-ray units must have exposure reproducibility, or the ability to duplicate certain radiographic exposures for any given combination of kVp, mA, and time.
- Exposure linearity is essential. When the mA is changed to a neighboring mA station, the most that linearity can vary is 10%.
- When screen-film image receptors are used, intensifying screens used in conjunction with matching radiographic film are predominantly rare earth screens. Carbon fiber is frequently used as a front material in a radiographic cassette.
- Radiographic grids increase patient dose in radiography; their use for examination of thicker body parts is a fair compromise because they remove scattered radiation emanating from the patient that would otherwise degrade the recorded image.
  - Because of increased sensitivity of photostimulable phosphor to scatter radiation before and after exposure to a radiographic beam, a grid may be used more frequently during computed radiography (CR) imaging. The use of a grid does increase patient dose but significantly improves radiographic contrast and visibility of detail.
- To limit the effects of inverse square falloff of radiation intensity with distance during a mobile radiographic examination, a source-to-skin distance (SSD) of at least 12 inches (30 cm) must be used.

---

*Bushong SC: *Radiologic science for technologists: physics, biology and protection*, ed 9, St. Louis, 2008, Mosby.

- With digital radiography, the latent image formed by x-ray photons on a radiation detector is actually an electronic latent image.* It is called a *digital image* because it is produced by computer representation of anatomic information. The image receptor is divided into small detector elements that make up the two-dimensional picture elements, or pixels, of the digital image. The pixels collectively produce a two-dimensional display of the information contained in a particular x-ray projection.† Radiographers must select correct technical exposure factors the first time to avoid overexposing patients when digital images are obtained.
- Computed radiography results when the invisible, or latent, image generated in conventional radiography is produced in a digital format using computer technology.
- The digital image can be displayed on a monitor for viewing, and it can be printed on a laser film when hard copy is needed.
- Fluoroscopic procedures produce the greatest patient radiation exposure rate in diagnostic radiology.
  - Minimize patient exposure time whenever possible.
  - Limit the size of the fluoroscopic field to include only the area of anatomy that is of clinical interest.
  - Employ the practice of intermittent, or pulsed, fluoroscopy to reduce the overall length of exposure.
  - Select the correct technical exposure factors to help minimize the amount of radiation received by a patient.
  - Ensure that the x-ray source-to-skin distance (SSD) is no less than 15 inches (38 cm) for stationary (fixed) fluoroscopes and no less than 12 inches (30 cm) for mobile fluoroscopes.
- During C-arm fluoroscopic procedures, the patient–image intensifier distance should be as short as possible.
- Cinefluorography can result in the highest patient doses of all diagnostic procedures.
  - Reduce patient dose by using intermittent activation of the fluoroscope to locate the catheter, limiting the time of the cine run, and using the last-image-hold feature to view the most recent image.
- During digital fluoroscopy the use of pulsed progressive systems lowers patient dose.
  - Use of the last-image-hold feature is another dose-reduction technique.
- High-level-control (HLC) fluoroscopy is used for interventional procedures.
  - The operating mode uses exposure rates that are substantially higher than those allowed for routine fluoroscopic procedures.
  - If skin dose in the range of 1 to 2 Gy (100 to 200 rad) is received, the Food and Drug Administration (FDA) requires that a notation be placed in the patient's record.
  - The radiographer generally has the responsibility for monitoring and documenting procedural fluoroscopic time when fluoroscopic equipment is used by nonradiologist physicians.

---

*Bushong SC: *Radiologic science for technologists: physics, biology, and protection*, ed 8, p. 589, St. Louis, 2004, Mosby.
†Seeram E: Digital image processing, *Radiol Technol* 75:6, 2004.

Exercise 1: Crossword Puzzle

Use the clues to complete the crossword puzzle.

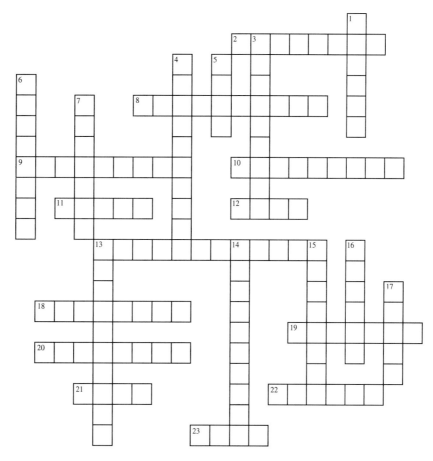

Down

1. Type of fluoroscopy that involves manual or automatic periodic activation of the fluoroscopic tube rather than lengthy or continuous activation.
3. Scientific term referring to the brightness of a surface.
4. Most versatile device for defining the size and shape of the radiographic beam.
5. Use of this device increases patient dose.
6. Type of cassette used for computed radiography.
7. Type of radiation that is reduced by the use of x-ray beam limitation devices.
13. Placed in the path of the x-ray beam to reduce exposure to the patient's skin and superficial tissues by absorbing most of the lower-energy photons from the heterogeneous beam.
14. Type of timer that must be provided and used with each fluoroscopic unit.
15. A device that electronically processes independent groups of information.
16. Miniature square boxes in the image matrix of a digital image.
17. What inherent plus added filtration equals.

Across

2. For diagnostic x-ray beams, half-value layer is expressed in millimeters of this material.
8. Type of image intensifier tubes found in the majority of image intensifiers.
9. Rare-earth phosphor that radiographic intensifying screens can be made of.
10. Quantity, or amount, of radiation.
11. Type of compensating filter that is attached to the lower rim of the collimator and positioned with its thickest part toward the toes and its thinnest toward the heel when obtaining a dorsoplantar projection of the foot.
12. Radiation-absorbent material used to make protective shielding.
13. Procedures that produce the greatest patient radiation exposure rate in diagnostic radiology.
18. Cone vision (daytime vision).
19. Mean energy of the x-ray beam.
20. Type of interventional procedure performed by a physician with the aid of fluoroscopic imaging.
21. What most radiation exposure in selective coronary arteriography results from.
22. Type of fiber material that is commonly used in the tabletop of a radiographic examining table.
23. Radiation (x-rays) emitted from parts of the tube other than the focal spot.

Exercise 2: Matching

Match the following terms with their definitions or associated phrases.

1. _____ inherent filtration
2. _____ HVL
3. _____ diagnostic-type protective tube housing
4. _____ spacer bars
5. _____ added filtration
6. _____ control panel
7. _____ scattered radiation
8. _____ PBL
9. _____ computed radiography (CR)
10. _____ radiographic beam defining system
11. _____ high-level-control fluoroscopy (HLCF)
12. _____ carbon fiber
13. _____ nit
14. _____ aperture diaphragm
15. _____ quantum mottle
16. _____ mobile (portable) x-ray unit

A. Equipment that should be used to perform radiographic procedures only on patients who cannot be transported to a fixed radiographic installation (an x-ray room)

B. A movie camera that uses either 16-mm or 35-mm film to record the image of the output phosphor of the image intensifier

C. Front material in a cassette that can result in a lower radiation dose for the patient because a lower radiographic technique is used to produce the recorded image

D. Device that increases the patient dose

E. Consists of two sets of adjustable lead shutters mounted within the collimator at different levels, a light source to illuminate the x-ray field and permit it to be centered over the area of clinical interest, and a mirror to deflect the light beam toward the patient to be radiographed

F. Feature of a radiographic collimator that automatically adjusts the collimator so that the radiation field size matches the film size

G. Allows the fluoroscopist to see the most recent image without exposing the patient to another pulse of radiation

H. The simplest of all beam-limitation devices

I. Thickness of a designated absorber (customarily a metal, such as aluminum) required to reduce the intensity (quantity or amount) of the primary beam by 50% of its initial value

J. Projects down from the x-ray tube housing to prevent the collimator from moving closer than 15 cm away from the patient

K. Sheets of aluminum (or its equivalent) of appropriate thickness localized outside the glass window of the x-ray tube housing above the collimator shutters

L. Required to protect the patient and imaging personnel from off-focus, or leakage, radiation by restricting the emission of x-rays to the area of primary beam

M. The distance from the anode focal spot to the radiographic image receptor

N. The glass envelope encasing the x-ray tube, the insulating oil surrounding the tube, and the glass window in the tube housing

O. Where technical exposure factors such as mA and kVp are selected and seen on indicators by the operator

P. Process in which the invisible, or latent image, generated in conventional radiography is produced in a digital format using computer technology; the digital image can be displayed on a monitor for viewing or printed on a laser film when hard copy is needed

17. _____ off-focus radiation
18. _____ last-image-hold feature for dose reduction
19. _____ digital radiography
20. _____ source-to–image receptor distance (SID)
21. _____ integral dose
22. _____ radiographic grid
23. _____ useful beam
24. _____ cinefluorography
25. _____ digital image

Q. An electronic latent image formed by x-ray photons on a radiation detector
R. Image produced by computer representation of anatomic information
S. A simple term for candelas per square meter
T. Term that is synonymous with stem radiation.
U. An operating mode of fluoroscopic equipment in which exposure rates are significantly higher than normally allowed for routine fluoroscopic procedures; this allows visualization of smaller and lower contrast objects than normally are visible during fluoroscopy
V. Product of dose and volume of tissue irradiated
W. Faint blotches (image noise) in the radiographic image produced by an intrinsic fluctuation in the incident photon intensity
X. Radiation that emerges directly from the x-ray tube collimator and moves without deflection toward a wall, door, viewing window, and so on
Y. All the radiation that arises from the interaction of an x-ray beam with the atoms of a patient or any other object in the path of the beam

Exercise 3: Multiple Choice

Select the answer that best completes the following questions or statements.

1. To meet radiation safety features, radiographic equipment must have a:
   1. Correctly functioning control panel
   2. Protective tube housing
   3. Radiographic examination table designed to reduce patient radiation dose
   A. 1 only
   B. 2 only
   C. 3 only
   D. 1, 2, and 3

2. There are various types of digital radiography image receptors. Some use a scintillator, such as amorphous silicon, to:
   A. Convert visible light into x-ray energy
   B. Convert x-ray energy into visible light
   C. Ensure adequate penetration of the anatomy to be imaged
   D. Reduce scattered radiation before it reaches the image receptor

3. The luminance of the collimator light source must be:
   A. Adequate to permit the localizing light beam to outline the margins of the radiographic beam adequately on the patient's anatomy
   B. Visible on the patient's anatomy only when all white light is turned off in the radiography room
   C. Less than 5 foot-candles
   D. At least 10 foot-candles

4. Which of the following results in an *increase* in the patient dose?
   A. Use of a radiographic grid
   B. Use of carbon fiber in the radiographic tabletop
   C. Use of rare earth intensifying screens with matching radiographic film
   D. Use of a variable rectangular collimator containing a spacer bar

5. The patient dose *decreases* and the life of the fluoroscopic tube *increases* with which of the following?
   A. Restriction of the fluoroscopic field to include only the area of clinical interest
   B. Use of a conventional fluoroscope rather than image intensification, or the use of digital fluoroscopy equipment
   C. Intermittent, or pulsed, fluoroscopy
   D. Darkness adaptation

6. When fluoroscopic field size is limited to include only the area of clinical interest by adequately collimating the x-ray beam, patient area or integral dose:
   A. Decreases substantially
   B. Increases substantially
   C. Remains the same as if the x-ray beam were not collimated
   D. Remains at zero

7. Digital radiography eliminates the need for almost all retakes resulting from improper technique selection because the image:
   A. Contrast and overall brightness can be manipulated after image acquisition
   B. Contrast and overall brightness cannot be manipulated after image acquisition
   C. Requires chemical processing to become visible
   D. Does not require chemical processing to become visible

8. Computed radiography involves:
   1. Use of conventional radiographic equipment
   2. Selection and use of standard technical exposure factors
   3. Traditional patient positioning performed by a radiographer
   A. 1 only
   B. 2 only
   C. 3 only
   D. 1, 2, and 3

9. Which of the following is the *most* versatile for defining the size and shape of the radiographic beam?
   A. Aperture diaphragm
   B. Radiographic cone shaped as a flared metal tube
   C. Radiographic cone shaped as a straight cylinder
   D. Light-localizing variable-aperture rectangular collimator

10. The use of digital radiographic systems offers a number of advantages over both CR and conventional film-screen systems. Some of these include:
    1. Immediate imaging results
    2. Lower dose
    3. Presence of a preinstalled grid
    A. 1 and 2 only
    B. 1 and 3 only
    C. 2 and 3 only
    D. 1, 2, and 3

11. In computed radiography imaging, when a grid is required to radiograph anatomy sections over 10 cm in thickness or for techniques that exceed 70 kVp, patient dose received is:
    A. About the same as with film-screen imaging because the same mAs is used
    B. Significantly higher than is delivered with film-screen imaging because the mAs required is significantly higher
    C. Significantly lower than is delivered with film-screen imaging because the mAs required is significantly lower
    D. Slightly lower than is delivered with film-screen imaging because the mAs required is slightly lower

12. Fluoroscopic equipment equipped with high-level control (HLC) may permit a skin entrance exposure rate *as great as* which of the following?
    A. 5 R/min ($5 \times 2.58 \times 10^{-4}$ C/kg/min)
    B. 10 R/min ($10 \times 2.58 \times 10^{-4}$ C/kg/min)
    C. 20 R/min ($20 \times 2.58 \times 10^{-4}$ C/kg/min)
    D. 50 R/min ($50 \times 2.58 \times 10^{-4}$ C/kg/min)

13. To protect the patient's skin from exposure to electrons produced by photon interaction with the collimator, the skin surface should be at least _____ *below* the collimator.
    A. 6 cm
    B. 12 cm
    C. 15 cm
    D. 20 cm

14. To reduce patient entrance dose during C-arm fluoroscopic procedures, the patient-image intensifier distance should be:
    A. As short as possible
    B. As long as possible
    C. Always set at a 40-inch SID
    D. Always set at a 72-inch SID

15. Which of the following may reduce patient exposure to off-focus radiation?
    A. Placing the second pair of shutters in the collimator below the level of the light source and mirror
    B. Placing the first pair of shutters in the collimator as close as possible to the x-ray tube window
    C. Transmitting an electric signal through the collimator's first and second pair of shutters
    D. Off-focus radiation in a collimator cannot be reduced.

16. Which of the following is an effective technique for reducing patient dose when a digital fluoroscopic system is used?
    A. Converting to non–image intensification fluoroscopy
    B. Increasing mAs significantly
    C. Using scotopic (rod) vision instead of photopic (cone) vision
    D. Using the last-image-hold feature

17. Compared with patients who undergo cinefluorographic procedures that use lower frame rates, patients who undergo more rapid dynamic function studies (e.g., heart catheterization) receive:
    A. Higher radiation doses
    B. Slightly lower radiation doses
    C. Significantly lower radiation doses
    D. Identical radiation doses

18. HLCF is an operating mode for state-of-the-art fluoroscopic equipment in which exposure rates are:
    A. Slightly higher than those normally allowed in routine fluoroscopic procedures
    B. Substantially higher than those normally allowed in routine fluoroscopic procedures
    C. Slightly lower than those normally used in routine fluoroscopic procedures
    D. Substantially lower than those normally used in routine fluoroscopic procedures

19. Monitoring and documentation of procedural fluoroscopic time is essential to good practice. The responsibility for monitoring and documentation generally belongs to:
    A. The nurse assisting the physician with the procedure
    B. The physician performing the fluoroscopic procedure
    C. The radiographer assisting with the procedure
    D. Radiology department secretarial personnel

20. HVL is expressed in:
    A. Centimeters of aluminum
    B. Centimeters of lead
    C. Millimeters of aluminum
    D. Millimeters of lead

21. Dose reduction and uniform imaging of body parts that vary considerably in thickness or tissue composition may be accomplished by use of:
    A. Compensating filters constructed of aluminum, lead-acrylic, or other suitable material
    B. Compensating filters constructed of lightweight plastic or wood
    C. Compensating filters made of carbon fibers
    D. Radiographic grids

22. Resolution of a digital image is sharper when pixels are:
    A. Larger
    B. Smaller
    C. Variable in size
    D. Variable in thickness

23. For certain radiographic examinations the use of asymmetric film emulsion and intensifying screen combinations results in a recorded image with:
    A. Greater uniformity and an increase in patient exposure
    B. Greater uniformity and a decrease in patient exposure
    C. Lesser uniformity and an increase in patient exposure
    D. Lesser uniformity and a decrease in patient exposure

24. Compared with the resolution of an optimal quality image produced on radiographic film, the resolution of a digital image is:
    A. Actually somewhat less
    B. Comparable to the quality of the imaged produced on radiographic film
    C. Actually somewhat greater
    D. Significantly greater

25. Some of the reasons for high exposures during interventional procedures include:
    1. The fluoroscopic tube being operated for longer periods of time in continuous and not pulsed mode
    2. Failure to use the protective curtain or floating shields on the stationary fluoroscopic equipment's image intensifier as a means of protection
    3. Extensive use of cine as a recording medium
    A. 1 and 2 only
    B. 1 and 3 only
    C. 2 and 3 only
    D. 1, 2, and 3

Exercise 4: True or False

Circle *T* if the statement is true; circle *F* if the statement is false.

1. T F State-of-the-art diagnostic radiographic and fluoroscopic equipment has been designed with many devices that radiologists and imaging personnel can use to optimize the quality of the image and also reduce radiation exposure for patients undergoing various imaging procedures.

2. T F It is acceptable for the radiographer to adjust the collimator so that the radiographic beam is slightly larger than the size of the image receptor.

3. T F Radiographic cones and aperture diaphragms are x-ray beam filtration devices.

4. T F When PBL is activated, the collimators are automatically adjusted so that the radiation field matches the size of the image receptor.

5. T F Inherent filtration in an x-ray tube used for routine radiography amounts to approximately 2.5 mm aluminum equivalent.

6. T F Because HVL is a measure of beam quality or the effective energy of the x-ray beam, a certain minimal HVL is required at a given peak kilovoltage.

7. T F Maintaining and enhancing subject contrast is not important in mammography.

8. T F Rare earth elements used in intensifying screens have high atomic numbers ranging from 80 to 95.

9. T F When operating a mobile radiographic unit, the radiographer must use an SID of at least 12 inches (30 cm) to limit the effects of the inverse square falloff of radiation intensity with distance.

10. T F In digital radiography the size of the pixels determines the sharpness of the image.

11. T F Barium platinocyanide is the most commonly used photostimulable phosphor used in computed radiography imaging plates.

12. T F Rare earth screens place less thermal stress on the x-ray tube, increasing its life span.

13. T F When rare earth screens are used, radiation shielding requirements for the x-ray room are increased because a general increase in x-radiation in the environment occurs.

14. T F The patient dose decreases as the grid ratio increases.

15. T F When a radiographic procedure is performed with a CR system, it is acceptable practice to overexpose a patient initially because the image obtained can be technically adjusted to acceptable quality, avoiding the possibility of repeat exposure for the patient.

16. T F In CR imaging the routine practice of overexposing patients to possibly avoid repeat radiographic exposures is ethical and acceptable.

17. T F It is possible that CR technique factors will be somewhat greater than those used in conventional radiography, in which 400 speed film-screen combinations are typically employed.

18. T F Correct matching of screen-film systems is essential; incorrectly matched or incompatible components can result in an increased patient dose.

19. T F Rare earth intensifying screens, which are made of rare earth phosphors (i.e., gadolinium, lanthanum, or yttrium), absorb approximately five times more x-ray energy than the previously used calcium tungstate screens; therefore they emit considerably more light, resulting in a significant reduction in the radiographic exposure required to obtain an image of acceptable quality.

20. T F The use of steel fiber as a front material in a cassette that holds radiographic film and intensifying screens is a recent technologic advancement.

21. T F Compared with conventional screen-film systems, the photostimulable phosphor in the CR imaging plate is much more sensitive to scatter radiation before and after it is sensitized through exposure to a radiographic beam. Because of this increase in sensitivity to scatter radiation, a radiographic grid may be used more frequently during CR imaging.

22. T F When compared with conventional screen-film systems, the photostimulable phosphor in the CR imaging plate is much less sensitive to scatter radiation before and after it is sensitized through exposure to a radiographic beam. Because of this decreased sensitivity, a radiographic grid may be used less frequently during CR imaging.

23. T F A primary protective barrier of 2 mm aluminum equivalent is required for an image intensifier unit.

24. T F The use of C-arm fluoroscopy in procedures such as surgical pinning of a fractured hip carries the potential for a relatively large patient radiation dose. C-arm fluoroscope operators, if standing close to the patient, may also be subjected to significantly increased occupational exposure in such cases.

25. T F Dose reduction techniques are especially important in cine because cine procedures can result in the highest patient doses of all diagnostic procedures. The high dose resulting from cine is caused by a relatively high inherent dose rate and the length of the procedure, particularly in cardiology, which involves cardiac imaging procedures such as heart catheterization, and in neuroradiology. Thus a percentage decrease in cine dose yields a greater actual dose reduction than the same percentage decrease in noncine procedures.

Exercise 5: Fill in the Blank

Using the following Word Bank, fill in the blanks with the word or words that best complete the statements.

center	federal	multifield
dead-man	image matrix	quality
decreases	incapacitated	quantum mottle
density	increase	reduces
distance	latitude	same
dose reduction	less	technique
electronic	limitation	under
energized	manufacturer	wedge
entrance	mAs	workstations
exit	mispositioning	

1. Although many safety features have been built into x-ray–producing machines by their _____ to ensure radiation safety, some features have also been included to meet _____ regulations.

2. Patient exposure can be substantially reduced by using appropriate beam _____ devices.

3. For dose reduction purposes, it is preferable to position the C-arm so that the x-ray tube is _____ the patient.

4. The fluoroscopic exposure control switch (e.g., the foot pedal) must be of the _____ type so that the exposure automatically terminates if the person operating the switch becomes _____.

5. Filtration _____ the overall intensity of the radiation.

6. Many quality assurance teams are now realizing that CR, because of its higher exposure _____, makes grid use on pediatric patients _____ necessary than was previously believed.

7. For the computer to correctly form a CR image, the body area or part being radiographed must be positioned in or near the _____ of the CR cassette.

8. _____ charts indicating optimal kVp for all CR projections should be available in the x-ray room near the operating console for the radiographer.

9. The _____ filter may be used to provide uniform density when the foot is radiographed in the dorsoplantar projection.

10. With digital radiography, the latent image formed by x-ray photons on a radiation detector is actually a(n) _____ latent image.*

11. Collimating to the anatomic area of interest has the _____ effect in cine as in ordinary fluoroscopy.

12. To limit the effects of inverse fall-off of radiation intensity with _____ during a mobile radiographic examination, an SSD of at least 12 inches (30 cm) must be used.

13. The numeric values of the digital image are aligned in a fixed number of rows and columns that form individual miniature square boxes, each of which corresponds to a particular place in the image. These boxes collectively constitute the _____ _____.

14. When using a radiographic grid, because some fraction of the image receptor is covered with lead, _____ must be increased to compensate for the use of this device.

15. Radiographic _____ is highest when scattered photons are not recorded on the image.

16. When compared with slower-speed rare earth film-screen image receptor systems, faster-speed rare earth film-screen image receptor systems can demonstrate an effect referred to as _____.

17. As kilovoltage increases, effective screen speed increases for rare earth screens, which _____ patient dose.

---

*Bushong SC: *Radiologic science for technologists: physics, biology and protection*, ed 8, St. Louis, 2004, Mosby.

18. If screen-film systems are not correctly matched or compatible, patient dose can _____.

19. In digital radiography the numeric value in each miniature square box that makes up the image matrix can be converted into a visual brightness, or _____ level, that can be seen on a video display monitor.

20. Digital radiographic images can be accessed at several _____ at the same time, making image viewing very convenient for physicians providing patient care.

21. Even though DR eliminates the need for almost all retakes resulting from improper technique selection, retake rates for reasons of _____ will not be affected.

22. Because an image intensification system greatly increases brightness, image intensification fluoroscopy requires less milliamperage than old-fashioned conventional fluoroscopy. The consequent decrease in exposure rate can result in a sizable _____ _____ for the patient.

23. Depending on their manufacturer and geographic location, _____ image intensification tubes vary in size, but the 25/17/12 cm (10/6.8/4.8 inch)–diameter trifield model may be the commercial tube most commonly used in general-purpose image intensification fluoroscopic units.

24. When the SSD is small (e.g., for mobile radiographic examinations), patient _____ exposure is significantly greater than _____ exposure. By increasing the SSD, the radiographer maintains a more uniform distribution of exposure throughout the patient.

25. When the enclosed phosphor of a CR cassette is exposed to x-rays, it becomes _____.

Exercise 6: Labeling

Label the following illustrations and table.

A. X-ray tube, collimator, and image receptor.

B. Image intensification fluoroscopic unit.

From Bushong SC: *Radiologic science for technologists: physics, biology and protection,* ed 9, St. Louis, 2008, Mosby.

C. HVL Required by the Radiation Control for Health and Safety Act of 1968 and detailed by the Bureau of Radiologic Health* in 1980

Peak Kilovoltage	Minimum Required HVL in Millimeters of Aluminum
30	1. _____
40	2. _____
50	3. _____
60	4. _____
70	5. _____
80	6. _____
90	7. _____
100	8. _____
110	9. _____
120	10. _____

*The Bureau of Radiological Health changed its name to the Center for Devices and Radiological Health in 1982.

Exercise 7: Short Answer

Answer the following questions by providing a short answer.

1. If adequate filtration of the radiographic beam were not present, how would the patient's radiation dose and the image process be affected?

_____

_____

2. Why is it impossible to eliminate all off-focus, or stem, radiation coming from the primary beam and exiting at various angles from the x-ray tube window?

3. Why is aluminum the metal most widely selected for filter material in general diagnostic radiology?

4. Why is a certain minimal HVL required at a given peak kilovoltage?

5. What should be done in DR imaging to hold technologists accountable for retakes necessitated by mispositioning?

6. During a fluoroscopic examination what benefits does the use of photopic, or cone, vision have for the radiologist?

7. What does inherent filtration include?

8. List three reasons for high radiation exposure during an interventional procedure performed by a physician who is not a radiologist.

9. According to the FDA recommendation, at what range of skin dose received from a fluoroscopic procedure should a notation be placed in a patient's record?

10. What is the advantage of using a pulsed progressive system for digital fluoroscopy?

11. How does filtration reduce the overall intensity of radiation in a radiographic beam? How does this affect the remaining photons in the beam?

12. With regard to the diagnostic x-ray tube, where is added filtration located?

13. What are the requirements for the construction of the x-ray tube housing?

14. Where must the control panel in a fixed radiographic room be located?

15. What requirement must be met by the thickness of a radiographic examination tabletop?

16. What is a synonymous term for a bilateral wedge filter?

17. List eleven procedures involving extended fluoroscopic time.

18. Why is a cumulative timing device needed on fluoroscopic equipment?

19. For dose reduction purposes, why is it best to position the C-arm of a C-arm fluoroscopic unit so that the x-ray tube is under the patient whenever possible?

_____

_____

20. To what do current federal standards limit entrance skin exposure rates of general-purpose intensified fluoroscopic units?

_____

_____

Exercise 8: General Discussion or Opinion Questions

The following questions are intended to allow students to express their knowledge and understanding of the subject matter or to present a personal opinion. The questions may be used to stimulate class discussion. Because answers to questions may vary, determination of the answer's acceptability is left to the discretion of the course instructor.

1. What radiation safety features may be found on state-of-the-art diagnostic radiographic and fluoroscopic equipment that will reduce patient radiation exposure?

2. During interventional fluoroscopic procedures, what strategies can be used to manage radiation dose to patients, x-ray equipment operators, and other staff?

3. What are the responsibilities of a radiographer who is working with a nonradiologist physician using a C-arm or stationary fluoroscope with HLC mode, while performing interventional procedures or other potentially lengthy tasks?

4. What radiation safety features may be found on state-of-the-art radiographic and fluoroscopic equipment that will reduce radiation exposure for the equipment operator?

5. With reference to radiation safety, compare film-screen technology with digital radiography.

POST-TEST

The student should take this test after reading Chapter 10, finishing all accompanying textbook and workbook exercises, and completing any additional activities required by the course instructor. The student should complete the post-test with a score of 90% or higher before advancing to the next chapter. (Each of the following 20 questions or blanks is worth 5 points.) Score = _____ %

1. Current federal standards limit entrance skin exposure rates of general-purpose intensified fluoroscopic units to a maximum of _____ R/min.

2. What type of material is commonly used in radiographic examination tabletops?

_____

3. Every diagnostic imaging system must have a _____ tube housing and a correctly functioning _____ panel.

4. What is the most versatile x-ray beam limitation device currently in use?

_____

5. Define *scattered radiation*.

   _____

   _____

6. How does the use of a radiographic grid affect the patient dose?

   _____

   _____

7. The numeric values of the _____ image are aligned in a fixed number of rows and columns that form individual miniature square boxes, each of which corresponds to a particular place in the image. These individual boxes collectively constitute the _____ _____.

8. Which of the following reduces patient exposure?
    1. Carbon fiber material in the front of a radiographic cassette
    2. Use of appropriate beam limitation devices
    3. Use of automatic collimation
   A. 1 and 2 only
   B. 1 and 3 only
   C. 2 and 3 only
   D. 1, 2, and 3

9. Filtration that includes the glass envelope encasing the x-ray tube, the insulating oil surrounding the tube, and the glass window in the tube housing is called:
   A. Added filtration
   B. Inherent filtration
   C. Total filtration
   D. HVL

10. When fluoroscopic field size is limited to include only the area of clinical interest by adequately collimating the x-ray beam, patient area or _____ _____ decreases substantially.

11. Compared with slower rare earth film-screen image receptors, faster rare earth film-screen image receptor systems can demonstrate an effect referred to as _____ _____.

12. For what type of procedures is high-level-control fluoroscopy used?

   _____

13. In computed radiography imaging, when a grid is required to radiograph anatomy sections over 10 cm in thickness or for techniques that exceed 70 kVp, patient dose received is significantly higher than is delivered with film-screen imaging because the _____ required is significantly higher.

14. What fluoroscopic practice should a radiologist use to reduce the overall length of the exposure for a given procedure?

   _____

   _____

15. To protect the patient's skin from exposure to electrons produced by photon interaction with the collimator, the skin surface should be at least _____ cm below the collimator.
    A. 3
    B. 5
    C. 10
    D. 15

16. During C-arm fluoroscopic procedures, what should the patient–image intensifier distance be?
    _____

17. In digital radiography the size of the _____ determines the sharpness of the image.

18. What must radiographic imaging equipment have so that the radiographer can determine how far the image receptor is from the anode focal spot?
    _____

19. Placing the first pair of shutters in the collimator as close as possible to the x-ray tube window may:
    A. Eliminate the need for a second pair of shutters
    B. Eliminate the need for added filtration
    C. Reduce patient exposure from the primary beam
    D. Reduce patient exposure from off-focus, or stem, radiation

20. In CR imaging the routine practice of overexposing patients to possibly avoid repeat radiographic exposures is _____ and _____.

11 Management of Patient Radiation Dose during Diagnostic X-Ray Procedures

Chapter 11 covers management of patient radiation dose during diagnostic x-ray procedures. A holistic approach to patient care is essential whenever such an x-ray procedure is in progress. This means treating the whole person rather than just the area of concern. Holistic patient care must begin with effective communication between the radiographer and patient. This type of dialogue alleviates the patient's uneasiness and increases the likelihood for cooperation and successful completion of the procedure. To take care of all patients appropriately, the reader should develop easily understandable communication skills.

Radiographers must limit the patient's exposure to ionizing radiation by employing appropriate radiation reduction techniques and by using protective devices that minimize radiation exposure. Patient exposure can be substantially reduced by using proper body or part immobilization, motion reduction techniques, appropriate beam limitation devices and adequate filtration of the x-ray beam, and gonadal or other specific area shielding. Selection of suitable technical exposure factors used in conjunction with either high-speed film-screen combinations or computer-generated digital images, correct radiographic film-processing techniques or appropriate digital image processing, and the elimination of repeat radiographic exposures can also contribute significantly to limiting patient exposure. Chapter 10 described and discussed imaging equipment, devices, and accessories that imaging professionals can use to reduce patient radiation exposure during diagnostic x-ray procedures. This chapter provides an overview of other methods and techniques that radiographers can also use to minimize the patient's exposure to radiation during radiologic examinations.

CHAPTER HIGHLIGHTS

- Effective communication with the patient is the first step in holistic patient care.
  - Imaging procedures should be explained in simple terms.
  - Patients must have an opportunity to ask questions and receive truthful answers within ethical limits.
- Adequate immobilization of the patient is necessary to eliminate voluntary motion.
  - Restraining devices are available to immobilize either the whole body or the individual body part to be radiographed.
  - Involuntary motion can be compensated for by shortening exposure time with an appropriate increase in mA and by using very-high–speed image receptors.
- Protective shielding may be used to reduce or eliminate radiation exposure to radiosensitive body organs and tissues.
  - The reproductive organs should be protected from exposure to the useful beam when they are in or within approximately 5 cm of a properly collimated beam, unless this would compromise the diagnostic value of the study.
  - Correctly placed, appropriate gonadal shielding can greatly reduce the radiation received by both sexes (50% reduction for females, 90% to 95% reduction for males).
- The clear lead shadow shield and a PA projection can significantly reduce the dose to the breast of a young patient undergoing a scoliosis examination.
- Appropriate technical exposure factors for each examination must be selected.
  - Techniques chosen should ensure a diagnostic image of optimal quality with minimal patient dose.
  - Standardized technique charts should be available for each x-ray unit to help provide a uniform selection of technical exposure factors. High kVp and lower mAs should be chosen whenever possible to reduce the amount of radiation received by the patient yet maintain acceptable radiographic contrast to ensure the presence of adequate information in the recorded image.
- Correct image processing techniques reduce radiographic exposure for patients by reducing the need for repeat examinations that result from poorly processed images.
  - Imaging departments should establish a quality control program to ensure standardization in film-processing techniques and processing of digital images.
- An air gap technique can be used as an alternative to the use of a grid.
- Repeat radiographic exposures must be minimized to prevent the patient's skin and gonads from receiving a double dose of radiation.
- Radiographic examinations should be performed only when the patient will benefit from useful information gained from the procedure. Nonessential radiologic examinations should not be performed.
- The amount of radiation received by a patient from diagnostic imaging procedures may be specified as entrance skin exposure (ESE), skin dose, gonadal dose, or bone marrow dose.
  - ESE is the easiest to obtain and most widely used.
  - The estimated genetically significant dose (GSD) for the population of the United States is about 0.20 mSv (20 mrem).

- A radiographer should carefully question female patients of childbearing age regarding any possibility of pregnancy before they undergo an x-ray examination.
    - If irradiation during an unknown pregnancy occurs, a calculated estimate of the approximate equivalent dose to the embryo-fetus as a result of the examination should be obtained.
- Nonpalpable breast cancer may be detected through mammography.
    - Federal regulations state that the mean dose to the glandular tissue of a 4.5-cm compressed breast using a screen-film mammography system should not exceed 3 mGy (300 mrad) per view.
    - Digital mammography units with the ability to enhance contrast with image gray level manipulation offers improvement for patients with dense breasts.
- CT scanning is considered a relatively high–radiation exposure diagnostic procedure because of increasing use of multislice spiral (helical) CT scanners using small slice thickness.
    - Skin dose and dose distribution are two concerns.
    - In spiral CT, patient dose is comparable with that of conventional CT when pitch ratio is about 1; patient dose is reduced when pitch is higher and increased when pitch is lower.
    - From a radiation protection point of view, the goal of CT imaging should be to obtain the best possible image while delivering an acceptable level of ionizing radiation to the patient.
    - The goal of the Alliance for Radiation Safety in Pediatric Imaging is to increase awareness of the need to reduce patient dose for pediatric patients, especially in CT imaging.
    - The Image Gently campaign advocates lowering patient dose by "child-sizing" the kV and mA, scanning only the indicated area, and removing multiphase scans from pediatric protocols.
- Children are much more vulnerable than adults to both the late somatic and genetic effects of ionizing radiation.
    - Use a PA projection to protect breasts of female patients.
    - In small girls, shielding of the ovaries requires shielding of the iliac wings as well as the sacral area when shielding is needed.
    - Adequate collimation of the radiographic beam to include only the area of clinical interest is essential, and effective immobilization techniques should be used when necessary. The use of a high mA station and short exposure time also helps to minimize patient motion.
- A developing embryo-fetus is especially sensitive to ionizing radiation.
    - Use the smallest technical exposure factors that will generate a diagnostically useful radiographic image, carefully collimate the beam to include only the anatomic area of interest, and cover the lower abdomen and pelvic region with a suitable contact shield if they do not need to be included in the examination.
    - "Abdominal radiological examinations that have been requested after full consideration of the clinical status of a patient, including the possibility of pregnancy, need not be postponed or selectively scheduled."[1]
    - Elective abdominal examinations of women of childbearing years should be performed during the first few days after the onset of menses to minimize the possible irradiation of an embryo.
    - A radiologic physicist should determine fetal dose if a pregnant patient is inadvertently irradiated.

Exercise 1: Crossword Puzzle

Use the clues to complete the crossword puzzle.

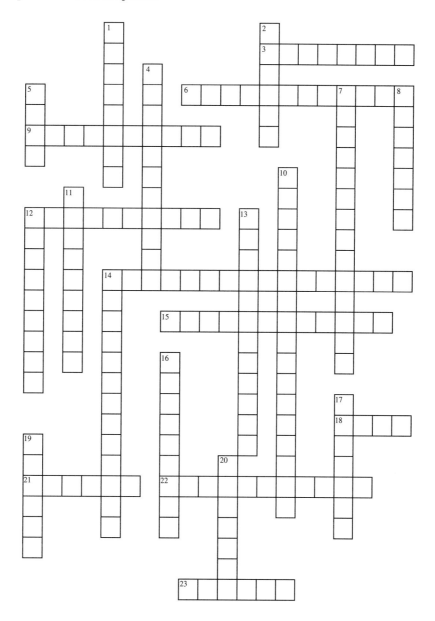

Down

1. Persons who are much more vulnerable than adults to both the late somatic and genetic effects of ionizing radiation.
2. A type of gonadal shield.
4. That which is extremely important in pediatric studies.
5. An air gap technique can be used as an alternative to the use of this device.
7. What is needed to eliminate or at least minimize patient motion?
8. Type of mammography units with the ability to enhance contrast with image gray level manipulation that offers improvement for dense breast patients.
10. Dosimeters that are the sensing devices most often used to measure skin dose directly.
11. When there is a lack of control, this type of motion results.
12. Person who should perform the calculations necessary to determine fetal exposure, if a pregnant patient is inadvertently irradiated.
13. The entrance exposure from a CT examination may be compared with the entrance exposure received during this routine type of examination.
14. Everyone within the imaging department should always behave as this type of professional.
16. Every imaging department should establish this type of written protocol for each of its radiologic procedures.
17. What the radiographic image will be if a patient moves during a radiographic exposure.

19. Type of patient shielding not typically used in CT.
20. Type of shielding used to protect male and female reproductive organs during a radiographic exposure.

Across

3. During a diagnostic x-ray procedure, this is the type of approach that is essential to patient care.
6. Type of technique charts that should be available for each x-ray unit to help provide a uniform selection of technical exposure factors.
9. Radiation that scatters from the CT slice being scanned into adjacent slices.
12. Type of shielding that may be used to reduce or eliminate radiation exposure to radiosensitive body organs and tissues.
14. Procedures that can result in the highest patient doses of all diagnostic procedures.
15. Patients with this potential should be shielded during x-ray procedures whenever the diagnostic value of the examination is not compromised.
18. Radiation-absorbent material used to make protective shielding.
21. Any image that must be performed more than once because of human or mechanical error during the production of the initial image.
22. Type of motion that can be compensated for by shortening exposure time with an appropriate increase in mA and by using very-high-speed-image receptors.
23. Type of fluoroscopy that involves manual or automatic periodic activation of the fluoroscopic tube by the fluoroscopist rather than lengthy continuous activation.

Exercise 2: Matching

Match the following terms with their definitions or associated phrases.

1. _____ body language
2. _____ external anatomic landmarks
3. _____ air gap technique
4. _____ flat contact shields
5. _____ referring physician
6. _____ gonadal shielding
7. _____ nonessential radiologic examinations
8. _____ epidermis
9. _____ double dose
10. _____ shaped contact shield
11. _____ bone marrow
12. _____ possibility of pregnancy
13. _____ gonadal dose

A. Standardization of film-processing techniques and processing of digital images, including monitoring and maintenance of all processing and image display equipment in a facility
B. Hangs over the area of clinical interest to cast a shadow in the primary beam over the patient's reproductive organs
C. Made of transparent lead-plastic material impregnated with approximately 30% lead by weight
D. Something that a radiographer should ask a female patient of childbearing age about before the patient undergoes an x-ray examination
E. Cup-shaped radiopaque device that encloses the scrotum and penis to protect the male reproductive organs from exposure to ionizing radiation
F. Individual picture element
G. Imaging procedure used to detect breast cancer that is not palpable in physical examinations
H. "An interaction that produces a satisfying result through an exchange of information"[2]
I. Promotes archival quality of the film whereby it will not deteriorate over time but will remain in its original condition
J. Areas on the patient that can be used to guide placement of a testicular or ovarian shield
K. Its primary function is to protect underlying tissues and structures
L. Alternative to using a radiographic grid to reduce scattered radiation during certain examinations
M. Individual responsible for ordering a radiologic examination

14. _____ effective communication

15. _____ mammography

16. _____ quality control program

17. _____ spiral CT

18. _____ clear lead shields

19. _____ entrance skin exposure (ESE)

20. _____ pixel

21. _____ genetically significant dose (GSD)

22. _____ elective x-ray examinations

23. _____ correct film processing

24. _____ shadow shield

25. _____ the Alliance for Radiation Safety in Pediatric Imaging

N. Unconscious actions, or nonverbal messages, that if understood as intended will promote effective communication between the radiographer and patient

O. Devices used during diagnostic x-ray procedures to protect the reproductive organs from exposure to the useful beam when they are in or within approximately 5 cm of a properly collimated beam

P. What the patient's skin and possibly the gonads receive whenever a repeat examination occurs

Q. Most frequently reported way to specify the amount of radiation received by a patient from a diagnostic imaging procedure

R. X-ray procedures that can be booked at an appropriate time to meet patient needs and safety

S. Radiation exposure received by the male and female reproductive organs

T. Their goal is to increase awareness of the need to reduce patient dose for pediatric patients especially in CT imaging

U. Type of computed tomography that presents a greater challenge for assessing patient dose than does conventional computed tomography

V. The equivalent dose to the reproductive organs that if received by every human would be expected to bring about an identical gross genetic injury to the total population, as does the sum of the actual doses received by exposed individual members of the population

W. X-ray studies performed in the absence of definite medical indications

X. Of great importance because it contains large numbers of stem, or precursor, blood cells that could be depleted or destroyed by substantial exposure to ionizing radiation

Y. Not suited for nonrecumbent positions or projections other than AP or PA

Exercise 3: Multiple Choice

Select the answer that *best* completes the following questions or statements.

1. Effective communication between the radiographer and the patient depends on which of the following?
   1. Verbal and nonverbal messages are congruent, so that they are understood as intended.
   2. The imaging procedure is explained in simple terms, and instructions are given clearly and concisely.
   3. The patient is given the opportunity to ask questions, which are answered truthfully within ethical limits.
   A. 1 only
   B. 2 only
   C. 3 only
   D. 1, 2, and 3

2. Interslice scatter during a CT scanning procedure results in which of the following?
   A. Decrease in patient dose
   B. Increase in patient dose
   C. Poorly defined cross-sectional image of the anatomy of interest
   D. Uniform distribution of radiation into all adjacent areas

3. Because no localizing light field exists and the field of view is usually moving during a fluoroscopic study:
   A. A flat contact shield is not suitable for use
   B. A shadow shield is not suitable for use
   C. A shaped contact shield is not suitable for use
   D. A shield that provides any type of gonadal protection is not suitable for use

4. Which of the following results in an *increase* in the patient dose?
   A. Use of the lowest possible kVp with the highest possible mAs for each examination
   B. Use of the correct radiographic film processing technique
   C. Use of standardized technique charts, when automatic exposure control is not used
   D. Use of the highest practicable kVp with the lowest possible mAs for each examination

5. In fluoroscopy, the amount of radiation that a patient receives is usually estimated by measuring the radiation exposure rate:
   A. At the tabletop and multiplying this by the kVp and mA used
   B. At the level of the Bucky tray and multiplying this by the kVp and mA used
   C. At the tabletop and multiplying this by the fluoro time
   D. At the level of the Bucky tray and multiplying this by the fluoro time

6. An optimal-quality cross-table lateral projection of the cervical spine was obtained using appropriate technical exposure factors and an 8:1 ratio grid. If another radiograph is obtained using an air gap technique and technical exposure factors that are comparable to those used with the 8:1 ratio grid, the patient dose is:
   A. About the same
   B. Significantly higher
   C. Significantly lower
   D. Not an issue because an air gap technique cannot be used in place of a grid for a lateral projection of the cervical spine

7. The skin and gonads of the patient receive a "double dose" of x-radiation:
   A. During all CT procedures
   B. Whenever an air gap technique is used
   C. Whenever gonadal shielding is used
   D. Whenever a repeat radiograph occurs as a consequence of human or mechanical error

8. The benefits of a repeat analysis program include:
   1. Increased awareness among staff and student radiographers of the need to produce optimal-quality recorded images
   2. Greater care in the production of radiographic images because radiographers are aware that the images are being reviewed
   3. Initiation and continuation of in-service education programs for imaging personnel covering problems or concerns identified through the program
   A. 1 only
   B. 2 only
   C. 3 only
   D. 1, 2, and 3

9. The exposure of the fetus to radiation arising from diagnostic procedures:
   A. Is not of concern because radiation from diagnostic procedures cannot cause any harm to an unborn fetus
   B. Will result in the immediate need for the patient to have a therapeutic abortion because of demise of the fetus from radiation exposure
   C. Would definitely be cause in all instances, by itself, for terminating a pregnancy
   D. Would rarely be cause, by itself, for terminating a pregnancy

10. When an individual of childbearing age undergoes a diagnostic x-ray procedure, gonadal shielding should be used to protect the reproductive organs from exposure to the useful beam:
    1. When the reproductive organs are in or within approximately 5 cm of a properly collimated x-ray beam
    2. Unless shielding will compromise the diagnostic value of the examination
    3. When the radiographer chooses to substitute gonadal shielding for adequate collimation of the x-ray beam
    A. 1 and 2 only
    B. 1 and 3 only
    C. 2 and 3 only
    D. 1, 2, and 3

11. Which of the following are *most often* used to assess skin doses?
    A. Compensating filters
    B. Filtration equivalent to 4 mm aluminum in the path of the x-ray beam
    C. Radiographic grids
    D. Thermoluminescent dosimeters

12. The Image Gently campaign advocates lowering patient dose by:
    1. Child-sizing the kV and mA
    2. Scanning only the indicated area
    3. Removing multiphase scans from pediatric protocols
    A. 1 only
    B. 2 only
    C. 3 only
    D. 1, 2, and 3

13. In computed tomography, which of the following factors affect(s) patient dose?
    1. Changes in noise level
    2. Pixel size
    3. Slice thickness
    A. 1 only
    B. 2 only
    C. 3 only
    D. 1, 2, and 3

14. If in the course of a specific radiographic procedure 75% of the active bone marrow were in the useful beam and were to receive an average absorbed dose of 0.4 mGy (40 mrad), the mean marrow dose would be which of the following?
    A. 0.3 mGy (30 mrad)
    B. 0.6 mGy (60 mrad)
    C. 0.9 mGy (90 mrad)
    D. 1 mGy (100 rad)

15. The actual dose delivered during a computed tomography scanning procedure depends on the:
    1. Amount of direct patient shielding used
    2. Type of scanner being used
    3. Radiation technical exposure factors selected
    A. 1 and 2 only
    B. 1 and 3 only
    C. 2 and 3 only
    D. 1, 2, and 3

16. Digital mammography units with the ability to enhance contrast with image gray level manipulation offers improvement for:
    A. All patients
    B. Patients with dense breasts
    C. Patients with less dense breasts
    D. Only patients with more aggressive breast cancer

17. To ensure a diagnostic image with minimal patient dose, the technique (technical exposure factors) chosen must ensure:
    1. Adequate radiographic density (exposure)
    2. An adequate amount of radiographic contrast between adjacent tissue densities
    3. Sufficient penetration of the area of clinical interest
    A. 1 only
    B. 2 only
    C. 3 only
    D. 1, 2, and 3

18. If a radiographic procedure will cause pain, discomfort, or any strange sensations, the patient:
    A. Must be informed before the procedure begins, but the radiographer should not overemphasize this aspect of the examination
    B. Must be informed before the procedure begins, and the radiographer should really stress this aspect of the examination
    C. Should not be informed before the procedure begins because he or she may decide not to have the procedure
    D. Should not be informed before the procedure begins so that he or she will not worry about this part of the examination

19. The product of x-ray electron tube current and the amount of time in seconds during which the x-ray beam is activated results in which of the following?
    A. kVp
    B. mA
    C. mAs
    D. HVL

20. Neglecting to use standardized technique charts when automatic exposure control (AEC) is not used necessitates estimating the technical exposure factors, which may result in:
    1. Poor-quality images
    2. Repeat examinations
    3. Unnecessary exposure for the patient
    A. 1 only
    B. 2 only
    C. 3 only
    D. 1, 2, and 3

21. Direct patient shielding is not typically used in:
    A. CR
    B. CT
    C. Diagnostic fluoroscopy
    D. Diagnostic radiography

22. From a radiation protection point of view, the goal of CT imaging should be to obtain the best possible image while delivering:
    A. An acceptable level of ionizing radiation to the patient
    B. As much ionizing radiation exposure as it will take to produce a perfect study
    C. As much ionizing radiation exposure as the patient can tolerate to produce the images
    D. Nonionizing radiation to produce the images of the patient

23. CT scanning is considered a relatively high–radiation exposure diagnostic procedure because of increasing use of:
    A. Contrast media
    B. Conventional CT scanners with higher pitch
    C. Multislice spiral (helical) CT scanners using small slice thickness
    D. CT scanners with tighter collimation

24. If a pregnant patient is inadvertently irradiated, which of the following medical professionals should determine fetal dose?
    A. Attending physician
    B. Administrator of the health care facility
    C. Radiologic physicist
    D. Radiologist

25. Which of the following radiographic procedures are considered unnecessary?
    1. Chest x-ray examination as part of a preemployment physical
    2. Chest x-ray examination for mass screening for tuberculosis
    3. Whole-body multislice spiral CT screening
    A. 1 and 2 only
    B. 1 and 3 only
    C. 2 and 3 only
    D. 1, 2, and 3

Exercise 4: True or False

Circle *T* if the statement is true; circle *F* if the statement is false.

1. T F Patient exposure can be substantially reduced by using proper body and/or part immobilization and motion reduction techniques.

2. T F Patients do not need to be given the opportunity to ask questions about their examination when they are having a routine x-ray procedure.

3. T F Poorly processed images on radiographic film will not deteriorate over time.

4. T F Shaped contact shields are not recommended for PA projections because the shield covers the anterior surface of the male reproductive organs and the x-ray beam enters from the posterior surface; therefore the shield does not protect the gonads.

5. T F An air gap technique removes scatter radiation by using a decreased object-to-image receptor distance.

6. T F With CR or DR, it is necessary to develop a policy whereby retaken image files can be recovered for analysis as part of a repeat analysis program.

7. T F The lens of the eye, the breasts, and the reproductive organs need not be selectively shielded from the useful beam.

8. T F Primary beam exposure for male patients may be reduced by only 25% when the gonads are covered with a contact shield containing 1 mm of lead.

9. T F To protect the ovaries of a female patient, the shield should be placed approximately 1 inch (2.5 cm) medial to each palpable anterior superior iliac spine.

10. T F The age recommendation for screening mammography is controversial because mammography is less accurate in the detection of breast cancer in younger women and likely to result in many false-positive readings, leading to unnecessary biopsies in that population.

11. T F Use of a lower peak kilovoltage (kVp) and a higher milliamperage and exposure time in seconds (mAs) reduces the patient dose.

12. T F The epidermis is composed of five layers.

13. T F Collimation should be a secondary protective measure, not a substitute for adequate gonadal shielding.

14. T F Dose reduction in mammography can be achieved by increasing the number of projections taken.

15. T F When a radiographic procedure is performed with a CR system, it is acceptable practice to overexpose a patient initially because the image obtained can be technically adjusted to acceptable quality, avoiding the possibility of repeat exposure for the patient.

16. T F Shielding of particularly sensitive breast tissue during a scoliosis examination may be accomplished using a clear lead shadow shield. The radiation dose to the breast of a young patient may be further reduced by performing the scoliosis examination with the x-ray beam entering the anterior surface of the patient's body instead of the posterior surface.

17. T F Poorly processed radiographs offer inadequate diagnostic information, leading to repeat examinations and unnecessary patient exposure.

18. T F Words and actions of medical imaging personnel must demonstrate understanding and respect for human dignity and individuality.

19. T F Inadequate or misinterpreted instructions may prevent the patient from being able to cooperate.

20. T F In mammography, axillary projections should be done routinely for all screening mammograms.

21. T F The dose distribution resulting from a CT scan is not the same as the dose distribution occurring in routine radiologic procedures.

22. T F In abdominal CT imaging, the entrance skin dose is approximately the same as the exit dose.

23. T F Patient dose decreases if CT technologists attempt to resolve smaller objects by setting thinner slice widths without sacrificing any SNR.

24. T F Because much evidence suggests that the developing embryo-fetus is especially radiation sensitive, special care is taken in radiography to prevent unnecessary exposure of the abdominal area of pregnant women.

25. T F The concept of genetically significant dose is used to assess the impact of gonadal dose.

Exercise 5: Fill in the Blank

Using the following Word Bank, fill in the blanks with the word or words that best complete the statements.

0.20 (20)	helical	poor
50	holistic	pregnancy
90	increases	protective
95	less	radiosensitive
additional	male	reduces
beam-defining	mean marrow	reduction
clinical interest	menstrual period	remote
computed tomography	milliampere-second	reproductive
cooperate	minimal	shadow
decreases	minimize	symphysis pubis
effective	over	
female	placement	

1. Radiographers must limit the patient's exposure to ionizing radiation by employing appropriate radiation _____ techniques and by using _____ devices that _____ radiation exposure.

2. _____ patient care must begin with _____ communication between the radiographer and the patient.

3. When patients understand the procedure and their responsibilities, they can more fully _____.

4. Repeat radiographic exposures sometimes can be attributed to _____ communication between the radiographer and the patient.

5. If gonadal shields are not placed correctly, the _____ organs will not be protected.

6. As a consequence of their anatomic location, the _____ reproductive organs receive about three times more exposure during a given radiographic procedure involving the pelvic region than do the _____ reproductive organs.

7. Specific area shielding for selective body areas other than the gonads significantly _____ radiation exposure to those areas and should be used whenever possible.

8. When a male patient is in the supine position, the _____ _____ can be used to guide shield placement over the testes.

9. Some fluoroscopic tubes are located above the patient and are referred to as _____ rooms because personnel set up the patient for the examination and then leave the room before activating the x-ray tube. In these rooms the shield should be placed _____ the patient.

10. The _____ light must be accurately positioned to ensure correct placement of the shadow shield.

11. When estimating approximate equivalent dose to the embryo-fetus, radiation output is specified in milliroentgens per _____.

12. _____ _____ is a frequently employed diagnostic x-ray imaging modality that is considered to be a relatively high radiation exposure examination.

13. As kVp _____ and mAs _____, radiographic contrast is reduced. Consequently, the amount of diagnostically useful information in the recorded image is reduced.

14. Adequate collimation of the radiographic beam to include only the area of _____ _____ is essential.

15. According to the U.S. Public Health Service, the estimated GSD for the population of the United States is about _____ mSv (_____ mrem).

16. Primary beam exposure for male patients may be reduced as much as _____% to _____% when the gonads are covered with a contact shield containing 1 mm of lead.

17. Suspended from above the radiographic beam–defining system, shadow shields hang over the area of clinical interest to cast a _____ in the primary beam over the patient's reproductive organs.

18. Selection of appropriate technical exposure factors for each x-ray examination is essential to ensure a diagnostic image with _____ patient dose.

19. For female patients, the placement of a flat contact shield containing 1 mm of lead over the reproductive organs reduces exposure by about _____%.

20. Occasionally it is permissible to obtain a _____ image, when recommended by the radiologist for the purpose of obtaining additional diagnostic information.

21. In simple terms the GSD concept suggests that the consequences of substantial absorbed doses of gonadal radiation become significantly _____ when averaged over an entire population rather than applied to just a few of its members.

22. Bone marrow dose may also be referred to as the _____ _____ dose.

23. The tight collimation of the CT beam makes possible its accurate _____ relative to the area of anatomy to be studied, which permits CT technologists to avoid exposing selected _____ organs, such as the eyes.

24. Spiral CT is also called _____ CT.

25. Whenever a female patient of childbearing age is to undergo an x-ray examination, it is essential that the radiographer carefully question the patient about the possibility of _____. Part of this questioning involves asking the patient for the date of her last _____ _____.

Exercise 6: Labeling

Label the following illustration and boxes.

A. Technical Exposure Factor Considerations
   1. _____
   2. _____
   3. _____
   4. _____
   5. _____
   6. _____
   7. _____

B. Lead filter with breast and gonad shielding device.

Courtesy Fluke Biomedical.

1. _____

2. _____

C. Benefits of a Repeat Analysis Program

1. _____

2. _____

3. _____

Exercise 7: Short Answer

Answer the following questions by providing a short answer.

1. How can radiographers limit the patient's exposure to ionizing radiation during a diagnostic x-ray procedure?

2. Why must the radiographer achieve a balance in technical radiographic exposure factors?

3. List four basic types of gonadal shielding devices that can be used during a diagnostic x-ray procedure.

4. When film-screen systems are used, what is the direct consequence of poorly processed radiographs?

5. What is protective shielding?

6. How is an air gap technique performed? How does use of this technique for certain examinations help reduce scattered x-rays? How does the patient dose received from an air gap technique compare with the dose received from use of a midratio grid?

7. What decision regarding the patient must the referring physician make before ordering a radiologic examination?

8. What are the five layers of the epidermis?

9. List four ways to specify the amount of radiation a patient receives from a diagnostic imaging procedure.

10. Why is direct patient shielding not typically used in CT?

11. What members of a population would be excluded from genetically significant dose considerations?

12. If a patient is to receive substantial pelvic irradiation and there is some doubt about her pregnancy status but there are no overriding medical concerns, what would be recommended before the pelvis is irradiated?

13. For women 50 years of age and older, how frequently do experts advise having a screening mammogram for early detection of breast cancer?

14. What is the benefit of good communication during a diagnostic x-ray procedure?

15. List six x-ray procedures that are now considered nonessential.

16. List seven categories that may be established for discarded images.

17. What are the two concerns related to patient dose in computed tomography scanning?

18. What is the first goal of the Alliance for Radiation Safety in Pediatric Imaging?

19. What does the Image Gently campaign include?

20. How are thermoluminescent dosimeters (TLDs) used to measure skin dose directly?

Exercise 8: General Discussion or Opinion Questions

The following questions are intended to allow students to express their knowledge and understanding of the subject matter or to present a personal opinion. The questions may be used to stimulate class discussion. Because answers to questions may vary, determination of the answer's acceptability is left to the discretion of the course instructor.

1. If a pregnant patient is irradiated inadvertently, what procedure should be followed?

2. Give examples of poor radiographer-patient communication, and explain in each situation how the radiographer could improve communication with the patient.

3. What are the benefits of the Alliance for Radiation Safety in Pediatric Imaging and the Image Gently campaign?

4. How do adults and children differ in terms of vulnerability to radiation exposure?

5. How does dose distribution resulting from a CT scan differ from the dose distribution occurring in routine radiologic procedures?

POST-TEST

The student should take this test after reading Chapter 11, finishing all accompanying textbook and workbook exercises, and completing any additional activities required by the course instructor. The student should complete the post-test with a score of 90% or higher before advancing to the next chapter. (Each of the following 20 questions or blanks is worth 5 points.) Score = _____ %

1. The _____ _____ _____ advocates lowering patient dose by "child-sizing" the kV and mA, scanning only the indicated area, and removing multiphase scans from pediatric protocol.

2. What is the current position of the American College of Radiology (ACR) regarding abdominal radiologic examinations that have been requested by a physician after full consideration of the clinical status of a patient, including the possibility of pregnancy?

3. Whenever a repeat radiograph must be taken as a consequence of human or mechanical error, the skin and gonads of the patient receive a _____ _____ of x-radiation.

4. What type of patient shielding is not typically used in computed tomography?

5. Define the term *genetically significant dose*.

6. To protect the ovaries of a female patient, where on the anatomy should an ovarian shield be placed?

7. When verbal messages and unconscious actions, or body language (i.e., nonverbal messages), are understood as intended, communication between the radiographer and patient is _____ .

8. Which of the following substantially reduces patient exposure?
    1. Use of proper body and/or part immobilization
    2. Use of appropriate technical exposure factors
    3. Use of gonadal or other specific area shielding
   A. 1 and 2 only
   B. 1 and 3 only
   C. 2 and 3 only
   D. 1, 2, and 3

9. Which of the following x-ray procedures are considered unnecessary?
    1. Chest x-ray examination as part of a preemployment physical
    2. Chest x-ray examination for mass screening for tuberculosis
    3. Whole-body multislice spiral CT screening
   A. 1 and 2 only
   B. 1 and 3 only
   C. 2 and 3 only
   D. 1, 2, and 3

10. Gonadal shielding should be a secondary protective measure, not a substitute for an adequately _____ beam.

11. Shielding of particularly sensitive breast tissue during a scoliosis examination may be accomplished using a clear lead shadow shield. The radiation dose to the breast of a young patient may be further reduced by performing the scoliosis examination with the x-ray beam entering the _____ surface of the patient's body instead of the _____ surface.

12. Who is responsible for ordering a diagnostic x-ray procedure?

13. Correctly placed, appropriate gonadal shielding can greatly reduce the exposure received by patients of both genders (_____ % for female patients, 90% to 95% for male patients).

14. According to the U.S. Public Health Service, what is the estimated GSD for the population of the United States?

15. Which of the following is a type of sensing device that is most often used to measure skin dose directly?
    A. Film badge
    B. OSL
    C. Pocket ionization chamber
    D. Thermoluminescent dosimeter

16. If irradiation of an unknown pregnancy occurs, what should be obtained?

17. Because of their anatomic location, the female reproductive organs receive about _____ times more exposure during a radiographic procedure involving the pelvic region than do the male reproductive organs.

18. What external anatomic landmark can a radiographer use for placement of a testicular shield on a male patient in the supine position?

_____

_____

19. Selection of appropriate technical exposure factors for each x-ray examination is essential to ensure a diagnostic image with
    A. Maximal patient dose
    B. Minimal patient dose
    C. No patient dose
    D. Selective organ dose only

20. Dose reduction in mammography can be achieved by limiting the number of _____ taken.

REFERENCES

1. Reynold FB: Prepared remarks for the October 20, 1976, American College of Radiology press conference.
2. Torres LS: *Basic medical techniques and patient care for radiologic technologists,* ed 5, Philadelphia, 1997, Lippincott Williams & Wilkins.

12 Management of Imaging Personnel Radiation Dose during Diagnostic X-Ray Procedures

Radiographers may be exposed to secondary radiation (scatter and leakage) while fulfilling professional responsibilities associated with diagnostic imaging. This increases their occupational exposure. Chapter 12 presents an overview of methods to reduce this exposure. Diagnostic x-ray suite protection design is also covered, with emphasis on new approaches to shielding in accordance with National Council of Radiation Protection and Measurements (NCRP) Report No. 147.

CHAPTER HIGHLIGHTS

- An annual occupational effective dose (EfD) of 50 mSv (5 rem) for whole-body exposure during routine operations and an annual EfD of 1 mSv (0.1 rem) for members of the general population has been established.
- A cumulative effective dose (CumEfD) limits a radiation worker's whole-body lifetime EfD to his or her age in years times 10 mSv (years × 1 rem).
- Radiation workers can receive a larger equivalent dose (EqD) than the general public without altering the genetically significant dose (GSD).
- Occupational exposure must be kept as low as reasonably achievable (ALARA).
- The following methods of reducing scatter radiation also reduce the occupational hazard for the radiographer:
  □ Use of beam-limitation devices, higher kVp and lower mAs techniques, appropriate beam filtration, and adequate protective shielding
  □ Correct use of protective apparel (e.g., lead aprons, gloves, thyroid shields)
  □ Reduction of repeat examinations
- The basic principles of time, distance, and shielding can be used to minimize occupational radiation exposure.
- Pregnant radiographers can wear an additional monitoring device at waist level to ensure that the monthly EqD does not exceed 0.5 mSv (0.05 rem).
- Primary and secondary protective barriers must be designed to ensure that annual EfD limits are not exceeded.
- To protect the radiographer and patient from leakage radiation, lead-lined metal diagnostic-type protective tube housing must be used.
- The following are required to protect the radiographer during routine fluoroscopy:
  □ The radiographer, in addition to wearing appropriate protective apparel, should stand as far from the patient as is practical and move closer to the patient only when assistance is required.
  □ A spot film device protective curtain and a Bucky slot shielding device must be used.
  □ The x-ray beam must be adequately collimated, and high-speed image receptor systems and a cumulative timing device should also be used.
- The following are required to protect the radiographer during mobile radiographic examinations:
  □ The radiographer must wear protective garments.
  □ The radiographer should stand at least 6 feet (1.8 m) from the patient, x-ray tube, and useful beam.
  □ The radiographer should stand at a right angle to the x-ray beam-scattering object (the patient) line.
- Limited exposure time and dose reduction features are required to protect the radiographer during high-level-control fluoroscopy.
- Distance is the most effective means of protection from ionizing radiation.
- If the peak energy of the x-ray beam is 100 kVp, a lead apron of at least 0.25 mm lead equivalent thickness should be worn if the radiographer cannot remain behind a protective barrier. A lead apron of 0.5 or 1 mm lead equivalent affords much greater protection.
- Lead gloves, a thyroid shield, and protective glasses sometimes are required.
- Radiographers should never stand in the primary beam to hold a patient during a radiographic exposure.
- When designing diagnostic x-ray suites, equivalent dose to radiation workers, nonoccupationally exposed personnel, and the general public must be taken into consideration.
  □ Facilities must be equipped with radiation-absorbent barriers.
  □ Occupancy factor, workload, and use factor must be considered during determination of thickness requirements for a protective barrier. Whether an area beyond a structure is designated as a controlled or an uncontrolled area is significant in determining the amount of radiation shielding to be added to that structure.
- Caution signs must be posted in any room or area where "radioactive materials or radiation sources are used or stored."*

---

*National Council on Radiation Protection and Measurements (NCRP): *Structural shielding design and evaluation for medical use of x-rays and gamma rays with energies up to 10 meV,* Report No. 49, Washington DC, 1976, NCRP.

Exercise 1: Crossword Puzzle

Use the clues to complete the crossword puzzle.

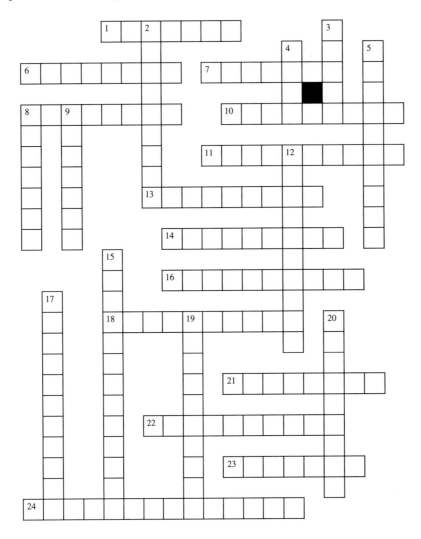

Down

2. The effect on the radiation dose as the length of exposure time decreases.
3. Accessory protective device made of lead-impregnated vinyl.
4. Scheduling radiographers to assigned clinical areas in a rotational pattern uses this cardinal principle as a means of radiation protection.
5. Use of this dose reduction material primarily benefits the patient.
8. Source of scattered radiation during a diagnostic x-ray procedure.
9. Type of secondary radiation.
12. The designation for an area adjacent to a wall of an x-ray room that is used only by occupationally exposed personnel.
15. How primary protective barriers are located in relation to the undeflected line of travel of the x-ray beam.
17. Term used when a technologist first informs her supervisor that she is pregnant.
19. Dose that is the product of the average absorbed dose in a tissue or organ in the human body and its associated radiation weighting factor, chosen for the type and energy of the radiation in question for radiation workers.
20. Type of protective barrier that a control-booth barrier is considered to be.

Across

1. One type of personal exposure that a radiographer's effective dose does not include.
6. The most effective means of protection from ionizing radiation.
7. A thickness of material that radiographers are not responsible for determining.
8. Established by most health care facilities to protect pregnant personnel from radiation.
10. Type of protective apparel that should be available for pregnant radiologists and radiographers.
11. Type of radiation-absorbent barriers such as walls and doors.
13. When it is not possible to use the cardinal principles of time or distance to minimize occupational exposure, this may be used to provide protection from radiation.
14. Type of radiation that poses the greatest occupational hazard in diagnostic radiology.
16. What a pregnant radiologic technologist must receive, after she informs a supervisor she is pregnant.
18. Type of eyeglasses that can be worn to reduce scattered radiation to the lenses of the eyes.
21. Quantity that best describes the weekly radiation use of a diagnostic x-ray unit.
22. Type of protective apron that can be worn for protection during pregnancy.
23. Radiation that emerges directly from the x-ray tube collimator.
24. A type of procedure that uses high-level-control fluoroscopy.

Exercise 2: Matching

Match the following terms with their definitions or associated phrases.

1. _____ 50 mSv (5 rem)
2. _____ control booth barrier
3. _____ 0.5 mSv (0.05 rem)
4. _____ ALARA concept
5. _____ diagnostic-type protective tube housing
6. _____ secondary radiation
7. _____ workload (W)
8. _____ spot film device protective curtain
9. _____ CumEfD limit
10. _____ occupancy factor (T)
11. _____ Bucky slot shielding device
12. _____ GSD
13. _____ inverse square law (ISL)
14. _____ use factor (U)

A. The intensity of radiation is inversely proportional to the square of the distance from the source.
B. Protects against leakage and scatter radiation.
C. Annual occupational effective dose for whole-body exposure during routine operations.
D. Possibility of developing a radiogenic cancer or the induction of a genetic defect as a consequence of radiation exposure.
E. Prevents direct, or unscattered, radiation from reaching personnel or members of the general public on the other side of the barrier.
F. Monthly allowable equivalent dose to the embryo-fetus from occupational exposure of a pregnant technologist.
G. Beam direction factor.
H. Annual EqD limit to localized areas of the skin and hands.
I. Specified in units of milliampere-seconds (mAs) per week or milliampere-minutes (mA-min) per week.
J. Automatically covers the Bucky slot opening in the side of the x-ray table during a standard fluoroscopic examination when the Bucky tray is positioned at the foot end of the table.
K. Required to protect both the radiographer and the patient from off-focus, or leakage, radiation by restricting the emission of x-rays to the area of the useful, or primary, beam.
L. Used to modify the shielding requirement for a particular barrier by taking into account the fraction of the work week during which the space beyond the barrier is occupied.
M. Permits the radiologist and assisting radiographer to remain outside the fluoroscopic room at a control console behind a protective barrier until needed.
N. Mode of operation in which the exposure rate may significantly exceed the rate used in routine fluoroscopy.

15. _____ scatter radiation

16. _____ protective eyeglasses

17. _____ secondary protective barrier

18. _____ high-level-control

19. _____ protective apparel

20. _____ remote control fluoroscopic system

21. _____ primary protective barrier

22. _____ C-arm fluoroscope

23. _____ 500 mSv (50 rem)

24. _____ occupational risk

25. _____ useful (primary) beam

O. Should be positioned between the fluoroscopist and the patient to intercept scattered radiation above the tabletop during a fluoroscopic examination.

P. A permanent protective barrier for the radiographer that is located in an x-ray room housing stationary (fixed) radiographic equipment.

Q. A radiation worker's whole-body lifetime effective dose must be limited to his or her age in years times 10 mSv (years × 1 rem).

R. All the radiation that arises from interactions of an x-ray beam with the atoms of an object in the path of the beam.

S. Principle that holds that occupational exposure of the radiographer and other occupationally exposed persons should be kept as low as reasonably achievable.

T. The average annual gonadal equivalent dose to members of the population who are of childbearing age.

U. The radiation that results from the interaction between primary radiation and the atoms of the irradiated object and the off-focus or leakage radiation that penetrates the x-ray tube protective housing; this radiation consists of scattered radiation and leakage radiation.

V. Glasses with optically clear lenses that contain a minimal lead equivalent protection of 0.35 mm.

W. X-rays emitted through the x-ray tube window or port.

X. Special garments (e.g., aprons, gloves, and thyroid shields) that conventionally are made of lead-impregnated vinyl and are worn during fluoroscopic and certain radiographic procedures.

Y. A portable device for producing real-time (motion) images of a patient; this device holds an x-ray tube at one end and an image intensifier at the other end; exposure of personnel is caused by scattered radiation from the patient.

Exercise 3: Multiple Choice

Select the answer that *best* completes the following questions or statements.

1. Because the workforce in radiation-related jobs is small compared with the population as a whole, the amount of radiation received by this workforce can be larger than the amount received by the general public without altering the:
   A. Genetically significant dose (GSD)
   B. Lethal dose (LD) 50/30
   C. Mean marrow dose (MMD)
   D. Tumor induction risk ratio (TIRR)

2. Which of the following is a tenet of the ALARA concept?
   A. The radiographer's occupational exposure should not exceed the annual EfD limit allowed for individual members of the general population.
   B. The radiographer's occupational exposure should be as high as necessary to allow for holding of patients during diagnostic x-ray procedures.
   C. The radiographer's occupational exposure for the whole body should limit that individual's lifetime EfD to his or her age times 50 mSv (years × 5 rem).
   D. The radiographer's exposure should be kept as low as reasonably achievable.

3. A facility that employs a pregnant diagnostic imaging staff member should provide that individual with an additional monitor to be worn at waist level during *all* radiation procedures. The purpose of this additional monitor is to ensure that the monthly EqD to the embryo-fetus does not exceed:
   A. 50 mSv (5 rem)
   B. 10 mSv (1 rem)
   C. 5 mSv (0.5 rem)
   D. 0.5 mSv (0.05 rem)

4. Which of the following are radiation sources that can be generated in a diagnostic x-ray room?
   1. Primary radiation
   2. Scatter radiation
   3. Leakage radiation
   A. 1 only
   B. 2 only
   C. 3 only
   D. 1, 2, and 3

5. During C-arm fluoroscopy, the exposure rate caused by scatter near the entrance surface of the patient (the x-ray tube side) _____ the exposure rate caused by scatter near the exit surface of the patient (the image intensifier side).
   A. Equals
   B. Exceeds
   C. Is slightly less than
   D. Is considerably less than

6. For high-level-control interventional procedures, the radiographer should verify that which of the following dose reduction features are available and in good working order?
   1. High-quality, low-dose fluoroscopy mode, and pulsed beam mode
   2. Collimation, optimal beam filtration, removable grids, variable optical aperture
   3. Roadmapping, time-interval differences, and last-image-hold mode
   A. 1 only
   B. 2 only
   C. 3 only
   D. 1, 2, and 3

7. In diagnostic radiology, which of the following radiation sources poses the *greatest* occupational hazard for the radiographer?
   A. Image-formation radiation
   B. Leakage radiation
   C. Primary radiation
   D. Scattered radiation

8. Which of the following methods and devices reduce(s) the radiographer's exposure during a fluoroscopic examination?
   1. Adequate x-ray beam collimation
   2. Control of technical exposure factors
   3. Use of a remote control fluoroscopic system
   A. 1 only
   B. 2 only
   C. 3 only
   D. 1, 2, and 3

9. If the peak energy of the diagnostic x-ray beam is 130 kVp, the primary protective barrier generally should consist of at least _____ and extend _____ upward from the floor of the x-ray room when the tube is 5 to 7 feet from the wall in question.
   A. 1/16-inch lead, 7 feet
   B. 1/16-inch lead, 10 feet
   C. 1/32-inch lead, 7 feet
   D. 1/32-inch lead, 10 feet

10. Which of the following radiation sources is the control booth barrier *not* intended to intercept in a diagnostic x-ray room?
    1. Leakage radiation
    2. Primary radiation
    3. Scattered radiation
    A. 1 only
    B. 2 only
    C. 3 only
    D. 1 and 3 only

11. Protective shielding for an uncontrolled area (e.g., a hall or corridor frequented by the general public) must ensure that the maximal EqD for that area is *no greater than* _____ per week.
    A. 1000 microsieverts (100 mrem)
    B. 100 microsieverts (10 mrem)
    C. 20 microsieverts (2 mrem)
    D. 10 microsieverts (1 mrem)

12. Which of the following statements is *true*?
    A. When wearing a protective apron, a radiographer may stand in the useful beam to restrain a patient during a difficult radiologic procedure.
    B. When wearing protective aprons, nurses, orderlies, relatives, or friends may stand in the useful beam to restrain a patient during a difficult radiologic procedure.
    C. When wearing protective aprons, pregnant radiographers or other nonoccupationally exposed pregnant women may stand in the useful beam to restrain a patient during a difficult radiologic procedure.
    D. Radiographers and nonoccupationally exposed individuals should never stand in the useful beam to restrain a patient during a radiographic procedure.

13. Of the devices listed below, which eliminates nonuseful low-energy photons from the primary beam?
    1. Collimator light source
    2. Electronic sensors
    3. Aluminum filtration
    A. 1 only
    B. 2 only
    C. 3 only
    D. 1, 2, and 3

14. Which of the following is the *most effective* means of protection from ionizing radiation normally available to the radiographer?
    A. Reducing the amount of time spent near a source of radiation
    B. Placing as much distance as possible between oneself and the source of radiation
    C. Remaining behind a mobile protective shield during an exposure
    D. Using protective shielding garments

15. The lead glass window of the control booth barrier in a stationary (fixed) radiographic installation typically consists of which of the following?
    A. 0.25 mm lead equivalent
    B. 0.5 mm lead equivalent
    C. 1 mm lead equivalent
    D. 1.5 mm lead equivalent

16. The beam direction factor is also known as the:
    A. Occupancy factor
    B. ISL
    C. Workload
    D. Use factor

17. If the intensity of the x-ray is inversely proportional to the square of the distance from the source, how does the intensity of the x-ray beam change when the distance from the source of radiation and a measurement point is quadrupled?
    A. It increases by a factor of 4 at the new distance.
    B. It increases by a factor of 16 at the new distance.
    C. It decreases by a factor of 16 at the new distance.
    D. It decreases by a factor of 4 at the new distance.

18. Leakage radiation and scatter radiation are forms of:
    A. Cosmic radiation
    B. Natural background radiation
    C. Nonionizing radiation
    D. Secondary radiation

19. Diagnostic x-ray installations must be equipped with:
    A. Barriers made of aluminum
    B. Barriers made of Sheetrock
    C. Radiation-absorbent barriers
    D. Radiation-nonabsorbent barriers

20. Which of the following principles can be used to minimize occupational radiation exposure?
    1. Time
    2. Distance
    3. Shielding
    A. 1 and 2 only
    B. 1 and 3 only
    C. 2 and 3 only
    D. 1, 2, and 3

21. Pregnant radiographers can wear an additional monitoring device at waist level to ensure that the monthly EqD does not exceed:
    A. 0.1 mSv (0.01 rem)
    B. 0.2 mSv (0.02 rem)
    C. 0.3 mSv (0.03 rem)
    D. 0.5 mSv (0.05 rem)

22. During fluoroscopy, which of the following will provide radiation protection for the radiographer and the radiologist?
    1. Adequate collimation of the x-ray beam
    2. Use of high-speed image receptor systems
    3. Use of a cumulative timing device
    A. 1 and 2 only
    B. 1 and 3 only
    C. 2 and 3 only
    D. 1, 2, and 3

23. Floors of radiation rooms except dental installations, doors, walls, and ceilings of radiation rooms exposed routinely to the primary beam are given a use factor of:
    A. 1
    B. ½
    C. ¼
    D. ¹⁄₁₆

24. If a radiographer stands 1 m from an x-ray tube and is subjected to an exposure rate of 4 mR/h, what will the exposure rate be if the same radiographer moves to a position 2 m from the x-ray tube?
    A. 1 mR/h
    B. 2 mR/h
    C. 8 mR/h
    D. 16 mR/h

25. If a radiographer moves closer to a source of radiation, the radiation exposure to the radiographer:
    A. Decreases slightly
    B. Decreases significantly
    C. Increases slightly
    D. Increases significantly

Exercise 4: True or False

Circle *T* if the statement listed below is true; circle *F* if the statement is false.

1. T F General fluoroscopy increases the radiographer's risk of exposure to ionizing radiation.

2. T F A radiographer's annual occupational EfD includes personal medical and natural background radiation exposure.

3. T F The ALARA concept takes economic and social factors into consideration.

4. T F Protective lead aprons and shielded barriers function as gonadal shields for diagnostic imaging personnel.

5. T F The intensity of radiation is directly proportional to the square of the distance from the source.

6. T F Clear lead-plastic overhead protective barriers used as an overhead x-ray barrier typically offer 2 mm lead equivalent protection.

7. T F If the peak energy of an x-ray beam is 100 kVp, a protective lead (Pb) apron must be equivalent to at least a 0.5-mm thickness of lead.

8. T F During a routine fluoroscopic examination, if the radiographer's immediate presence is not required near the x-ray table to assist the radiologist, the radiographer may stand behind the radiologist, who is wearing protective apparel.

9. T F The spot film device protective curtain protects the radiologist and radiographer at the gonadal level.

10. T F For C-arm devices with similar fields of view, the dose rate for personnel located within a meter of the patient is comparable to that in routine fluoroscopy—approximately several milligrays (mGy) per hour.

11. T F The physical configuration of a C-arm fluoroscopic unit allows for many methods of achieving protection from scattered radiation.

12. T F From the perspective of increased radiation safety, it is best to reverse the C-arm to place the x-ray tube under the table and the image intensifier over the table.

13. T F A radiographer may hold a patient during a radiographic exposure as long as the radiographer stands in the useful beam.

14. T F In a typical x-ray suite, the most common primary radiation barrier is that behind the wall Bucky unit.

15. T F Because scatter and leakage radiation emerge in all directions in the x-ray room, every wall, door, viewing window, and other surface are always struck by some quantity of radiation.

16. T F Filtration primarily benefits the radiographer.

17. T F During a diagnostic x-ray procedure, the patient becomes a source of scattered radiation as a consequence of the coherent scattering process.

18. T F At a 90-degree angle to the primary x-ray beam, at a distance of 1 m (3.3 feet), the scattered x-ray intensity is generally approximately 1/1000 of the intensity of the primary x-ray beam.

19. T F Methods and techniques that reduce patient exposure also reduce exposure for the radiographer.

20. T F Pregnant diagnostic imaging department staff members must immediately stop performing their respective duties and discontinue employment as a consequence of pregnancy.

21. T F The amount of radiation a worker receives is inversely proportional to the length of time the individual is exposed to ionizing radiation.

22. T F If a declared-pregnant radiographer is reassigned to a lower–radiation exposure risk area, other unknowing potentially pregnant radiographers can be subject to increased risk. Therefore the declared-pregnant radiographer does not necessarily need to be reassigned to a lower–radiation exposure area as a direct consequence of the declared pregnancy.

23. T F In accordance with ALARA guidelines, work schedules are designed to evenly distribute radiation exposure risk to all employees.

24. T F In a typical x-ray room, a secondary barrier should overlap the primary barrier by about ½ inch (1.25 cm).

25. T F During a fluoroscopic examination, a radiographer need not wear a protective apron.

Exercise 5: Fill in the Blank

Using the following Word Bank, fill in the blanks with the word or words that best complete the statements.

1/16 inch	Compton scatter (term may be used more than once)	patient
1/32 inch		perpendicular
0.05		reduction
0.5 (term may be used more than once)	decrease	right angles
	distance (term may be used more than once)	routine
0.25 mm	equivalent dose	safety
0.5 mm (term may be used more than once)	four (term may be used more than once)	scattered (term may be used more than once)
1 mm	gloves	shielding (term may be used more than once)
2.1	high-tension	shortening
5	housing	thyroid shields
7	increased	time
90	least	wraparound
aprons	magnify	
assistance		

1. Although the radiographer and other diagnostic imaging personnel are allowed to absorb more radiation than the general public, the _____ _____ received must be minimized whenever possible.

2. _____ radiation poses the greatest occupational hazard in diagnostic radiology.

3. Correct radiographic film processing techniques lead to a _____ in the number of repeat examinations required, with a resultant _____ in exposure to the radiographer.

4. After receiving radiation safety counseling, a pregnant radiologic technologist must read and sign a form acknowledging that she has received counseling and understands the ways to implement appropriate measures to ensure the _____ of the embryo-fetus.

5. If a declared-pregnant radiographer is reassigned to a lower–radiation exposure risk area, other unknowing potentially pregnant radiographers can be subject to _____ risk.

6. _____ the length of time spent in a room where x-radiation is produced reduces occupational exposure.

7. The most effective means of protection from ionizing radiation is _____.

8. Structural barriers such as walls and doors in an x-ray room provide radiation _____ for both imaging department personnel and the general public.

9. Accessory protective shielding includes _____, _____, and _____ made of lead-impregnated vinyl.

10. No one should touch the tube _____ or _____ cables while a radiographic exposure is in progress.

11. When high-speed image receptor systems are used, smaller radiographic exposure (less milliamperage) is required, which results in fewer x-ray photons being available to produce _____ _____. Because of this reduction in _____ _____, personnel exposure is decreased.

12. It is imperative that the EqD to the embryo-fetus from occupational exposure of the mother not exceed the NCRP-recommended monthly EqD limit of _____ mSv (_____ rem) or a limit of _____ mSv (_____ rem) during the entire pregnancy.

13. Maternity protective aprons consist of _____ lead equivalent over their entire length and width and also have an extra _____ lead equivalent protective panel that runs transversely across the width of the apron to provide added safety for the embryo-fetus.

14. Shortening the length of _____ spent in a room where x-radiation is produced, standing at the greatest _____ possible from an energized x-ray beam, and interposing a radiation-absorbent _____ material between the radiation worker and the source of radiation all reduce occupational exposure.

15. When the distance from the x-ray target, a point source of radiation, is doubled, the radiation at the new location spans an area _____ times larger than the original area. However, because the same amount of radiation exists to cover this larger area, the intensity at the new distance decreases by a factor of _____.

16. Primary protective barriers are located _____ to the undeflected line of travel of the x-ray beam.

17. If the peak energy of the x-ray beam is 130 kVp, the primary protective barrier in a typical installation consists of _____ lead and extends _____ feet (____ m) upward from the floor of the x-ray room when the x-ray tube is 5 to 7 feet from the wall in question.

18. In a typical diagnostic x-ray installation, the secondary barrier consists of _____ lead.

19. During fluoroscopy and x-ray special procedures, a neck and thyroid shield can guard the thyroid area of occupationally exposed people. It should be _____ lead equivalent.

20. To ensure protection from _____ radiation emanating from the patient during a fluoroscopic examination, the radiographer should stand as far from the _____ as is practical and should move closer to the patient only when _____ is required.

21. Protective lead gloves of at least _____ lead equivalent should be worn whenever the hands must be placed near the fluoroscopic field.

22. For better visualization of small body parts, C-arm fluoroscopes have the capability to _____ the image.

23. A _____ protective apron is recommended to protect personnel who must move around the x-ray room during a fluoroscopic examination.

24. The radiographer should attempt to stand at _____ _____ (____ degrees) to the x-ray beam-scattering object (the patient) line; when the protective factors of distance and shielding have been accounted for, this is the place where the _____ amount of scattered radiation is received.

25. In _____ imaging, because the image contrast and overall brightness can be manipulated after image acquisition, the need for almost all retakes resulting from improper technique selection is eliminated.

Exercise 6: Labeling

Label the following illustrations.

A. Relationship between distance and intensity.

B. Protective barriers.

C. Standing at right angles to the scattering object.

Exercise 7: Short Answer

Answer the following questions by providing a short answer.

1. With what occupational groups are monitored diagnostic imaging personnel compared for the purpose of assessing occupational risk?

2. From what types of x-radiation are lead aprons designed to provide protection?

3. How does the use of high-speed imaging receptor systems help reduce occupational exposure for x-ray personnel?

4. Why should a pregnant radiographer "declare" a pregnancy?

5. List the three basic principles of radiation protection.

6. Who should determine the exact requirements for protective structural shielding for a particular imaging facility?

7. Protective aprons, gloves, and thyroid shields are made of what material?

8. How can scattered radiation to the lens of the eyes of diagnostic imaging personnel be substantially reduced?

9. How does a lead-lined, metal, diagnostic-type protective tube housing protect the radiographer and the patient from off-focus, or leakage, radiation?

10. How does the use of a remote control fluoroscopic unit increase the safety of imaging personnel?

11. From the perspective of increased radiation safety, why is it best to place the x-ray tube end of the C-arm under the table and the image intensifier over the table whenever possible?

12. During operating room procedures in which cross-table exposures are obtained with a mobile C-arm fluoroscope, where is the potential for scatter dose lower in relation to the patient?

13. How can the radiologist or other interventional physician reduce radiation exposure during a high-level-control interventional procedure?

14. Why should physicians performing interventional procedures wear extremity monitors? What is the annual EqD limit for localized areas of the skin and hands? What can physicians use to protect their hands during an interventional procedure?

15. List eight radiation-absorbent barrier-design considerations.

Exercise 8: Discussion or Opinion Questions

The following questions are intended to allow students to express their knowledge and understanding of the subject matter or to present a personal opinion. The questions may be used to stimulate class discussion. Because answers to these questions may vary, determination of the answer's acceptability is left to the discretion of the course instructor.

1. Of what importance is protective structural shielding in an imaging facility? What factors must be considered in planning structural shielding? Who is responsible for the planning of such structural shielding?

2. What are some of the requirements for posting caution signs to alert others of the presence of radioactive materials or radiation areas? What do these signs look like?

3. What types of protective apparel are usually available for personnel in most health care facilities? Give examples of appropriate use of each of these items in a clinical setting.

4. When performing a mobile radiographic examination, what radiation protection problems can a radiographer encounter? How can each problem be safely resolved?

5. When operating a mobile C-arm fluoroscope in the operating room during a surgical procedure, what radiation protection problems may a radiographer encounter? How can each problem be safely resolved?

Exercise 9: Calculation Problems

Solve the following problems.

The inverse square law expresses the relationship between distance and intensity (quantity) of radiation and governs the dose received. The law states, "The intensity of radiation is inversely proportional to the square of the distance from the source." To be more precise, as the distance between the radiation source and a measurement point increases, the quantity of radiation measured at the more distant position decreases by the square of the ratio of the original distance from the source to the new distance from the source.

This decrease in radiation intensity physically occurs because the area, which the same flux of x-rays at the original location now covers at the new location, has increased by the square of the relative distance change. For example, as demonstrated in the sample problem that follows, when the distance from the x-ray target, a point source of radiation, is doubled, the radiation at the new location spans an area four times larger than the original area. However, because the same amount of radiation exists to cover this larger area, the intensity at the new distance consequently decreases by a factor of four.

The ISL may be stated as a formula, shown in the following equation. A mathematical example is also provided.

$$\frac{I_1}{I_2} = \frac{(d_2)^2}{(d_1)^2}$$

I_1 expresses the exposure (intensity) at the original distance; I_2 expresses the exposure (intensity) at the new distance; d_1 expresses the original distance from the source of radiation; and d_2 expresses the new distance from the source of radiation.

Example: If a radiographer stands 2 m from an x-ray tube and is subjected to an exposure rate of 6 mR/h, what will the exposure rate be if the same radiographer moves to a position 4 m from the x-ray tube?

Answer:

$$\frac{I_1}{I_2} = \frac{(d_2)^2}{(d_1)^2}$$

$$\frac{6}{I_2} = \frac{(4)^2}{(2)^2}$$

$$\frac{6}{I_2} = \frac{16}{4} \text{ (cross multiply)}$$

$$16\, I_2 = 24$$

$$I_2 = 1.5\, mR/hr$$

1. If a radiographer stands 3 m from an x-ray tube and is subjected to an exposure rate of 9 mR/h, what will the exposure rate be if the same radiographer moves to a position 6 m from the x-ray tube?

2. If a radiographer stands 2 feet from an x-ray tube and is subjected to an exposure rate of 5 mR/h, what will the exposure rate be if the same radiographer moves to a position 4 feet from the x-ray tube?

3. If a radiographer stands 5 m from an x-ray tube and is subjected to an exposure rate of 4 mR/h, what will the exposure rate be if the same radiographer moves to a position 10 m from the x-ray tube?

4. If a radiographer stands 1 m from an x-ray tube and is subjected to an exposure rate of 7 mR/h, what will the exposure rate be if the same radiographer moves to a position 2 m from the x-ray tube?

5. If a radiographer stands 6 feet from an x-ray tube and is subjected to an exposure rate of 6 mR/h, what will the exposure rate be if the same radiographer moves to a position 12 feet from the x-ray tube?

6. If a radiographer stands 2 m from an x-ray tube and is subjected to an exposure rate of 6 mR/h, what will the exposure rate be if the same radiographer moves to a position 6 m from the x-ray tube?

The ISL also implies that if a radiographer moves closer to a source of radiation, radiation exposure of the radiographer drastically increases.

Example: If a radiographer stands 1 foot from an x-ray source instead of 6 feet, the radiographer's exposure increases by a factor of $(6/3)^2 = 4$.

$$6 \div 3 = 2$$

$$2 \times 2 = 4$$

7. If a radiographer stands 5 m from an x-ray source instead of 10 m, the radiographer's exposure increases by a factor of _____.

8. If a radiographer stands 4 feet from an x-ray source instead of 12 feet, the radiographer's exposure increases by a factor of _____.

9. If a radiographer stands 1 m from an x-ray source instead of 4 m, the radiographer's radiation exposure increases by a factor of _____.

10. If a radiographer stands 2 feet from an x-ray source instead of 8 feet, the radiographer's radiation exposure increases by a factor of _____.

POST-TEST

The student should take this test after reading Chapter 12, finishing all accompanying textbook and workbook exercises, and completing any additional activities required by the course instructor. The student should complete the post-test with a score of 90% or higher before advancing to the next chapter. (Each of the following 20 questions or blanks is worth 5 points.) Score = _____ %

1. What is the most effective means of protection from ionizing radiation?

2. Most health care facilities have policies for protecting pregnant personnel from radiation. Under these policies an imaging professional who becomes pregnant first informs her supervisor. After this voluntary _____ has been made, the health care facility officially recognizes the pregnancy.

3. Define the term *genetically significant dose*.

4. What poses the greatest occupational hazard for the radiographer in diagnostic radiology?

5. Protective lead aprons and shielded barriers function as _____ shields for diagnostic imaging personnel.

6. State the ISL.

7. Radiographers and nonoccupationally exposed individuals should never stand in the useful beam to _____ a patient during a radiographic procedure.

8. What are the three basic principles of radiation protection?

9. Primary protective barriers are located:
    A. At a 45-degree angle to the undeflected line of travel of the x-ray beam
    B. At a 60-degree angle to the undeflected line of travel of the x-ray beam
    C. Parallel to the undeflected line of travel of the x-ray beam
    D. Perpendicular to the undeflected line of travel of the x-ray beam

10. A neck and thyroid shield can guard the thyroid area of occupationally exposed people during general fluoroscopy and x-ray special procedures. It should be:
    A. 1 mm lead equivalent
    B. 0.5 mm lead equivalent
    C. 0.25 mm lead equivalent
    D. 0.1 mm lead equivalent

11. For most mobile radiographic units that are not remote controlled, the cord leading to the exposure switch must be long enough to permit the radiographer to stand at least _____ from the patient, the x-ray tube, and the useful beam.
    A. 3 feet
    B. 6 feet
    C. 9 feet
    D. 12 feet

12. During high-level-control fluoroscopic interventional procedures, _____ should be kept so that the cumulative fluoroscopic exposure time may be determined.

13. When determining _____ requirements for a protective barrier, occupancy factor, workload, and use factor must be considered.

14. A spot film device protective curtain, or sliding panel, of a minimum thickness of 0.25 mm lead equivalent normally should be positioned between the fluoroscopist and the patient to intercept _____ radiation above the table top.

15. If a radiographer stands 3 m from an x-ray tube and is subject to an exposure rate of 10 mR/h, what will the exposure rate be if the same radiographer moves to a position 6 m from the x-ray tube?

16. What type of protective barrier is needed to protect personnel against scatter and leakage radiation?

17. If the image intensifier of a mobile C-arm fluoroscope is positioned as close to the _____ as possible, the required fluoroscopic x-ray beam intensity is minimized.

18. What does the NCRP currently recommend as an annual EqD limit to localized skin and hands?

19. Methods and techniques that reduce patient exposure also reduce exposure for the

20. It is imperative that the EqD to the embryo-fetus from occupational exposure of the mother not exceed the NCRP-recommended monthly EqD limit of _____ mSv (_____ rem) or a limit of 5 Sv (0.5 rem) during the entire pregnancy.

13 Radioisotopes and Radiation Protection

Chapter 13 covers radioisotopes and radiation protection. This chapter provides a brief description of the use of radioisotopes in both diagnostic and therapeutic medical procedures and discusses some relevant radiation safety issues. It also focuses on the use of radiation as a terrorist weapon and includes some fundamental principles for dealing with radioactive contamination in a health care setting.

CHAPTER HIGHLIGHTS

- Isotopes are atoms that have the same number of protons within the nucleus but have different numbers of neutrons.
  - Some nuclei of isotopes have too many neutrons or too many protons.
  - Radioactive isotopes spontaneously undergo changes or transformations to rectify their unstable arrangement.
- Rapidly dividing cells that are well oxygenated are very radiosensitive.
  - When cells are radiosensitive, cancerous growths or tumors can be eliminated or at least controlled by irradiation of the area containing the growth.
- Therapeutic isotopes may be characterized by relatively long half-lives.
- Fast electrons are beta radiation.
- Gamma rays and x-ray photons differ only in their point of origin.
- Iodine-125 decays with a half-life of 59.4 days by a process called *electron capture*.
- The most practical radiation protection to follow for patients having therapeutic prostate seed implants is use of the concepts of distance and time.
- The radioactive isotope strontium-89 (^{89}Sr) is a bone-seeker.
- A neutrino is a particle that has almost negligible mass and no electric charge but carries away any excess energy from the nucleus of the atom.
- When iodine-131 is being administered to treat a hospitalized patient for thyroid cancer, a large, up to 1-inch thick, rolling lead shield can be positioned between the patient and any attending personnel for protection.
- Diagnostic techniques in nuclear medicine typically make use of short-lived radioisotopes as radioactive tracers.
  - Technetium-99m is the most common radioisotope used in nuclear medicine.
- Positron emission tomography (PET) makes use of annihilation radiation events.
  - When annihilation occurs, the positron and electron interact destructively and annihilate each other. Their respective masses convert into energy that will be carried off by two photons emerging from the annihilation site in opposite directions, each with a kinetic energy of 511 keV.
  - Fluorine-18 is the most important isotope used for PET scanning.
  - PET is an important imaging modality because it can examine metabolic processes within the body.
  - Fluorodeoxyglucose (FDG) is a radioactive tracer that is taken up or metabolized by cancerous cells and that will reveal their location through positron emission decay and subsequent generation of oppositely traveling annihilation photons.
  - A PET/CT scanner can detect the presence of regions of abnormally high glucose metabolism, providing evidence that there is metastasis to other body areas, and at the same time can obtain detailed information about the location and size of these lesions or growths.
  - Positron emitters result in the production of high-energy radiation, and for this reason, design of a PET/CT imaging suite involves significant radiation safety concerns.
- Most hospitals have radiation emergency plans for handling emergency situations involving radioactive contamination.
- A radioactive dispersal device, or *dirty bomb,* is a radioactive source mixed with conventional explosives, the actual long-term health effects of which will most likely be minimal.
  - If radioactive material from a dirty bomb remains in a small area, few people may be affected.
  - On the other hand, if enough explosives are used to spread the radioactive material over a broad area, the radioactivity will be diluted and may not be much higher than background levels.
  - If a dirty bomb were to explode with the same force as the explosion at Chernobyl, the actual number of radiation injuries could be quite small.
- The United States currently has emergency responders who are prepared and equipped to monitor and assess personnel exposure on site in an emergency situation.
  - After explosion of a dirty bomb, externally contaminated individuals can be decontaminated by removal of contaminated clothing and immersion in a shower.
  - Geiger-Müller (GM) detectors may be used by trained emergency personnel to monitor contamination levels.
  - During an emergency situation, individuals engaged in nonlifesaving activities are to work under a dose limit of 50 mSv (5 rem) per event; persons performing lifesaving activities have a dose limit of 250 mSv (25 rem).

- If surface contamination is suspected, emergency personnel should protect themselves by wearing gowns, masks, and gloves while working with the patient.
- Handling of patients with internal contamination will vary, depending on the clinical and radiologic form of contamination. Strategies may include dilution and blocking absorption in the gastrointestinal tract. Potassium iodide can be administered to block further uptake of radioactive iodine in the thyroid gland.

Exercise 1: Crossword Puzzle

Use the clues to complete the crossword puzzle.

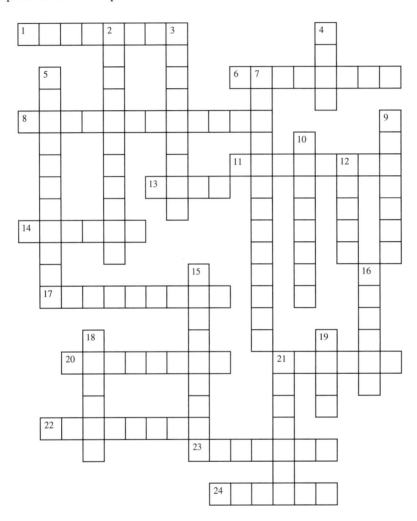

Down

2. Type of isotopes that are characterized by relatively long half-lives.
3. Element that has the same chemical properties as calcium.
4. Type of radiation that fast electrons are.
5. Where radioactive tablets dissolve in the human body.
7. Used in nuclear medicine to detect the spread of cancer into bone.
9. Type of energy possessed by two photons emerging from an annihilation site.
10. A well-designed PET/CT scanning facility will take good advantage of this powerful radiation protection tool.
12. If a wound contains radioactive material, this procedure is usually sufficient to decontaminate the area to allow medical personnel to provide medical attention.
15. What it may be to monitor all workers involved in a radiation emergency.
16. One item that personnel should wear when working with a patient who has received radioactive surface contamination.
18. Type of public concern that the explosion of a dirty bomb will become.
19. Level of energy that annihilation photons emanating in all directions from the patient having a PET/CT scan study possess.
21. Form of ordinary sugar that the radioactive tracer FDG is similar to in chemical behavior.

Across

1. For a patient with radiation sickness, the aspect that medical management should be geared to treat during the first 48 hours after exposure.
6. Gland in which iodine-125 seeds may be implanted for therapeutic purposes.
8. Condition of clothing that would need to be removed during the process of radioactive decontamination.
11. Positively charged electron.
13. After an explosion of a dirty bomb, this radioactive material will contaminate some individuals.
14. Point where gamma rays and x-rays differ.
17. Type of processes in the human body examined by positron emission tomography.
20. Table that lists the elements.
21. Counter that is used to monitor radioactive contamination.
22. Surface contamination.
23. Gland where sodium iodide (^{123}I) will preferentially concentrate.
24. Type of significant radiation concerns that PET/CT imaging suites involve.

Exercise 2: Matching

Match the following terms with their definitions or associated phrases.

1. _____ PET/CT scanner
2. _____ radiation emergency plan
3. _____ beta decay
4. _____ decontamination
5. _____ Environmental Protection Agency (EPA)
6. _____ half-value layer (HVL)
7. _____ radioisotopes
8. _____ radioactive contamination
9. _____ ^{18}F
10. _____ surface contamination
11. _____ neutrino
12. _____ annihilation radiation
13. _____ proton
14. _____ nuclear medicine

A. An electrically neutral particle that is believed to have almost negligible mass.
B. Dirty bomb.
C. Process wherein an inner-shell electron is captured by one of the nuclear protons, followed directly by the two combining to produce a neutron.
D. Atoms that have the same number of protons within the nucleus but have different numbers of neutrons.
E. Byproduct of the pair production interaction.
F. Radioactive tracer compound that is very similar in chemical behavior to ordinary glucose and therefore will be taken up or metabolized by cancerous cells, and it also will reveal their locations through its positron emission decay and subsequent generation of oppositely traveling annihilation photons.
G. Modality that uses ionizing radiation for the treatment of disease—namely, cancer.
H. Isotopes of a particular element that are unstable because of their neutron-proton configuration.
I. Modality that produces axial images by making use of annihilation radiation that is initiated by the radioactive decay of the nucleus of an unstable isotope.
J. Removal of radioactive material from an area or from clothing or a person.
K. Process by which a nucleus relieves instability through transformation of a neutron into a combination of a proton and an energetic electron (called a *beta particle*), and the emission of another particle called a *neutrino*.
L. Branch of medicine that uses radioisotopes to study organ function, to detect the spread of cancer into bone, and to treat certain types of disease.
M. U.S. government agency that facilitates the development and enforcement of regulations controlling radiation in the environment; it sets limits for radioactive contamination that assume that a 1-in-10,000 risk of causing a fatal cancer is unacceptable.
N. Radioactive isotope used for PET scanning.

15. _____ isotopes
16. _____ FDG
17. _____ electron capture
18. _____ neutron
19. _____ computed axial tomography (CAT)
20. _____ positron
21. _____ Geiger-Müller (GM) detector
22. _____ kinetic energy
23. _____ radiation therapy
24. _____ PET
25. _____ radioactive dispersal device

O. Radioactive material that is attached to or associated with dust particles or is in liquid form on various surfaces.
P. Process by which a computer-reconstructed transverse (or axial) image of a patient is created by an x-ray tube detector assembly rotating 360 degrees about a specific part of the body.
Q. Energy of motion.
R. A device that detects individual radioactive particles or photons and that also serves as the primary radiation survey instrument for area monitoring in nuclear medicine facilities.
S. A unit that is physically joined in a tandem configuration with a CAT scanner to produce a one-joint imaging device. Using FDG ^{18}F, it can detect abnormally high regions of glucose metabolism, which are evidence of the spread of cancer or of metastatic disease in other body areas. It also provides detailed information about the location and size of these lesions or growths.
T. The thickness of a designated absorber required to reduce the intensity of the primary beam by 50% of its initial value.
U. A positively charged electron, which is a form of antimatter.
V. A plan hospitals can implement for handling emergency situations involving radioactive contamination.
W. External contamination of the skin or clothing with radioactive material.
X. An electrically neutral particle found in the nucleus of the atom; one of the fundamental constituents of the atom.
Y. One of the three main constituents of an atom, it carries a positive electrical charge.

Exercise 3: Multiple Choice

Select the answer that *best* completes the following questions or statements.

1. Isotopes are atoms that have the *same* number of _____ in the nucleus but have *different* numbers of _____.
   A. electrons, protons
   B. neutrons, electrons
   C. protons, neutrons
   D. protons, neutrinos

2. Which two terms are synonymous?
   A. X-rays and gamma rays
   B. Alpha rays and beta rays
   C. Fast electrons and beta rays
   D. Neutrons and neutrinos

3. Which of the following radioisotopes used in radiation therapy is considered a bone-seeker?
   A. ^{125}I
   B. ^{125}Te
   C. ^{131}I
   D. ^{89}Sr

4. A particle that has almost negligible mass and no electric charge but carries away any excess energy from the nucleus of the atom is a(n):
   A. Electron
   B. Neutron
   C. Neutrino
   D. Proton

5. The branch of medicine that uses radioisotopes to study organ function, to detect the spread of cancer into bone, and to treat certain types of disease is:
   A. Chemotherapy
   B. Computed radiography
   C. Nuclear medicine
   D. Ultrasonography

6. The radioisotope *most often* used in nuclear medicine diagnostic studies is:
   A. ^{125}I
   B. ^{131}I
   C. ^{89}Sr
   D. ^{99m}Tc

7. PET makes use of what radiation events?
   A. Annihilation radiation
   B. Compton scattering
   C. Photodisintegration
   D. Photoelectric interaction

8. During the process of annihilation, the positron and the electron annihilate each other and their rest masses are converted into energy, which appears in the form of two 511-keV photons, each moving:
   A. At exactly a 45-degree angle to the other
   B. In the same direction
   C. In opposite directions
   D. Toward the nucleus of the original atom

9. The isotope *most often* used in PET scanning is:
   A. ^{60}Co
   B. ^{18}F
   C. ^{131}I
   D. ^{89}Sr

10. Positron emitters result in the production of:
    A. High-energy radiation
    B. Intermediate-energy radiation
    C. Low-energy radiation
    D. No radiation

11. Most hospitals have _____ for handling emergency situations involving radioactive contamination.
    A. No radiation emergency plans
    B. No trained personnel
    C. Radiation emergency plans and trained personnel
    D. A and B

12. A 1-in-10,000 probability of causing a fatal cancer corresponds to an effective dose of approximately
    A. 1 mSv (100 rem)
    B. 2 mSv (200 rem)
    C. 3 mSv (300 rem)
    D. 5 mSv (500 rem)

13. For exposures localized to *specific* regions of the body, medical management involves
    1. Prevention of infection
    2. Control of pain
    3. Possibly skin grafts
    A. 1 and 2 only
    B. 1 and 3 only
    C. 2 and 3 only
    D. 1, 2, and 3

14. The physical half-life of ^{18}F is
    A. 10 min
    B. 110 min
    C. 10 years
    D. 110 years

15. ^{125}I is an unstable isotope of the element iodine with:
    A. 73 protons and 102 neutrons
    B. 102 protons and 73 neutrons
    C. 53 protons and 72 neutrons
    D. 72 protons and 53 neutrons

16. The design of a PET/CT imaging suite involves:
    A. No radiation safety concerns
    B. Minimal radiation safety concerns
    C. Moderate radiation safety concerns
    D. Significant radiation safety concerns

17. Each _____ nuclear transformation by positron decay yields two highly penetrating 511-keV photons.
    A. ^{18}Cl
    B. ^{18}F
    C. ^{18}I
    D. ^{18}Sr

18. In beta decay a neutron transforms itself into a combination of:
    A. A positron and an alpha particle
    B. A positron and a negatron
    C. A proton and an energetic electron
    D. A proton and an alpha particle

19. Radioactive ^{89}Sr is a:
    A. Bone evader
    B. Bone demineralizer
    C. Bone mineralizer
    D. Bone seeker

20. Fast electrons are:
    A. Alpha radiation
    B. Beta radiation
    C. Gamma radiation
    D. X-radiation

21. A neutrino is a particle that has almost _____ mass and _____ electric charge but carries away any excess energy from the nucleus of the atom.
    A. significant, positive
    B. significant, negative
    C. negligible, no
    D. negligible, positive

22. Gamma rays and x-ray photons only differ in their:
    A. Wavelength
    B. Position on the electromagnetic spectrum
    C. Point of origin
    D. Energy and frequency

23. If a dirty bomb were to explode with the same force as the explosion at the Chernobyl nuclear power station in 1986, the actual number of injuries attributed to radiation exposure could be:
    A. Catastrophic
    B. Enormous
    C. Quite small
    D. Nonexistent

24. Potassium iodide may be administered to block further uptake of radioactive iodine in the:
    A. Gallbladder
    B. Liver
    C. Kidneys
    D. Thyroid gland

25. The thickness of a designated absorber required to reduce the intensity of the primary beam by 50% of its initial value defines:
    A. Radioisotope shielding barrier equivalent
    B. Lead apron thickness requirement
    C. HVL
    D. Positron emission

Exercise 4: True or False

Circle *T* if the statement is true; circle *F* if the statement is false.

1. T F ^{125}I is a stable isotope.

2. T F Distance and time are the best radiation safety practices for therapeutic implants such as the ^{125}I seed implant for the prostate gland.

3. T F Hospital rooms for ^{131}I patients usually are isolated and carefully prepared with absorbent cloths to substantially minimize radiation exposure to personnel and visitors from emitted gamma radiation from the patient or from contaminated surfaces.

4. T F In a PET device, annihilation radiation is initiated by the radioactive decay of the nucleus of a stable atom.

5. T F The nucleus of ^{18}F has 18 neutrons.

6. T F The possible use of radiation as a terrorist weapon is of no concern to the general population.

7. T F If radioactive material from a dirty bomb remains in a small area, few people might be affected.

8. T F Because monitoring of all workers involved in a radiation emergency may be difficult, a dose rate criterion often is used.

9. T F The same procedures that control infection are not useful for preventing the spread of radioactive contamination.

10. T F Diagnostic techniques in nuclear medicine typically make use of long-lived radioisotopes as radioactive tracers.

11. T F ^{131}I is the radioisotope most often used in nuclear medicine.

12. T F ^{89}Sr is a pure beta emitter.

13. T F Neutrinos almost never interact in matter and are therefore nearly impossible to detect.

14. T F In the United States, emergency responders are equipped to monitor and assess personnel exposure on site in an emergency situation.

15. T F Most hospitals stock cutie pies to monitor radiation contamination levels during an emergency.

16. T F Radiation therapy uses ionizing radiation for the radiologic diagnosis of disease.

17. T F Radioactive contamination may consist of surface, internal (inhaled or ingested), internal wound, or external wound contamination.

18. T F A positron is a normal form of matter.

19. T F ^{123}I undergoes radioactive decay by the process of electron capture, with an average half-life of 13.3 hours.

20. T F ^{99m}Tc is an extremely versatile radioisotope because it can be incorporated into a wide variety of different compounds or biologically active substances, each with a specificity for different tissues or organs.

21. T F Each ^{18}F nuclear transformation by positron decay yields two highly penetrating 511-keV photons, which can be shielded by an ordinary lead apron.

22. T F ^{18}F has a physical half-life of 110 min; therefore the patient's degree of radioactivity declines naturally throughout the preparation time, with approximately 25% to 30% lost by the time of scanning.

23. T F The only cases of acute radiation syndrome at Chernobyl were among emergency workers, primarily firemen who worked very near the reactor.

24. T F A dirty bomb is unlikely to cause contamination with so much radioactive material that a victim could not receive medical attention.

25. T F Removal of surface radioactive contamination involves removal of the patient's clothing and the use of a shower to cleanse the skin.

Exercise 5: Fill in the Blank

Using the following Word Bank, fill in the blanks with the word or words that best complete the statements.

6 (term may be used more than once)	full	positron
9	Geiger	pregnant
90	isolated	prep
adjacent	metabolic	radiation
annihilation	metastasis	radiosensitive
beta	minimize	radiotracer
calcium	monitoring	residual
dirty bomb	nucleus	sparing
electron capture	patient	unstable
	plastic container	vary

1. For ^{125}I seed implants, the goal is to deliver 145 Gy to at least _____% of the prostate's volume while limiting the radiation dose as much as possible to _____ structures such as the urethra, bladder, and anterior rectal wall.

2. For cancer patients in whom other methods of treatment have failed and who now have _____ to bone, infusion of ^{89}Sr delivers radiation therapy to those areas.

3. ^{99m}Tc has a half-life of _____ hours and decays by emission from its _____, primarily of gamma ray photons of 140-keV energy.

4. _____ emitters produce high-energy radiation.

5. Every patient who is to have a PET/CT scan requires _____ time.

6. After the attack on the World Trade Center on September 11, 2001, the possibility of the use of other possible terrorist weapons, such as _____, became a public health concern.

7. A radioactive source mixed with conventional explosives describes a radioactive dispersal device, or _____ _____.

8. Rapidly dividing cells that are well oxygenated are very _____.

9. Fast-moving electrons are called _____ radiation.

10. ^{125}I decays with a 59.4 half-life process called _____ _____.

11. During administration of iodine-131 to treat a hospitalized patient for thyroid cancer, a large, up to 1-inch thick, rolling lead shield can be positioned between the _____ and any attending personnel for protection.

12. Radioactive isotopes spontaneously undergo changes or transformations to rectify their _____ arrangement.

13. PET makes use of _____ radiation events.

14. PET is an important imaging modality because it can examine _____ processes in the body.

15. _____ counters can be used by trained emergency personnel to monitor radioactive contamination levels.

16. Handling of patients with internal contamination will _____, depending on the clinical and radiologic form of contamination.

17. Clothing that has been contaminated with radioactive material should be placed in a _____ _____ and set aside for later evaluation.

18. ^{125}I patients should significantly limit the duration of close contact (less than 3 feet [1 m]) with small children and _____ women for _____ months after the implant procedure.

19. Strontium and _____ are members of the same family of elements in the periodic table.

20. For a patient who has thyroid cancer, it is desirable to strongly irradiate any _____ thyroid tissue not removed by surgery while significantly _____ surrounding tissue and other organs.

21. Hospital rooms for ^{131}I therapy patients usually are _____ and carefully prepared with absorbent cloths to substantially _____ radiation exposure to both personnel and visitors from gamma radiation emitted from the patient or from contaminated surfaces.

22. ^{123}I is a _____ compound.

23. The nucleus of ^{18}F has _____ neutrons.

24. A well-designed PET/CT facility is arranged so that no areas of _____ occupancy are adjacent to a high-energy radiation source.

25. _____ of all radiation workers involved in a radiation emergency may be difficult.

Exercise 6: Labeling
Label the following table.

A. Dose-effect relationship after acute whole-body radiation from gamma rays or x-rays*

Whole-Body Absorbed Dose	Effect
0.05 Gy	No symptoms
1. ____	No symptoms, but possible chromosomal aberrations in cultured peripheral-blood lymphocytes
2. ____	No symptoms (minor decreases in white blood cell and platelet counts in a few persons)
3. ____	Nausea and vomiting in approximately 10% of persons within 48 hr after exposure
4. ____	Nausea and vomiting in approximately 50% of persons within 24 hr, with marked decreases in white blood cell and platelet counts
5. ____	Nausea and vomiting in 90% of persons within 12 hr, and diarrhea in 10% within 8 hr; 50% mortality in the absence of medical treatment
6. ____	100% mortality within 30 days because of bone marrow failure in the absence of medical treatment
7. ____	Approximate dose that is survivable with the best medical therapy available
8. ____	Nausea and vomiting in all persons in less than 5 min; severe gastrointestinal damage; death likely in 2-3 wk in the absence of treatment
9. ____	Cardiovascular collapse and central nervous system damage, with death in 24-72 hr

*Gusev I, Guskova AK, Mettler FA Jr, eds: *Medical management of radiation accidents*, ed 2, Boca Raton, Fla, 2001, CRC Press.

Exercise 7: Short Answer
Answer the following questions by providing a short answer.

1. How are therapeutic isotopes characterized?

_____

_____

2. How does electron capture occur?

_____

_____

3. How does beta decay occur?

4. What type of radioisotopes are typically used in nuclear medicine as radioactive tracers? How do these radionuclides work?

5. Why is PET an important imaging modality?

6. What benefit does the radioactive tracer FDG provide in PET imaging?

7. What benefit is obtained by combining PET and CT into one imaging device, called a *PET/CT scanner?*

8. What event led to the possibility of radiation being used as a terrorist weapon?

9. Why does the EPA set limits for radioactive contamination?

10. If a patient has surface radioactive contamination, what protective apparel should personnel wear?

11. Besides trained emergency personnel, who would be available to assess radioactive contamination in a health care facility during a radiation emergency?

12. How do personnel adhere to normal badge limits during a radiation emergency?

13. Describe the medical management of a patient during the first 48 hours of treatment for acute radiation syndrome.

14. What is annihilation radiation?

15. What is a radioactive dispersal device?

Exercise 8: General Discussion or Opinion Questions

The following questions are intended to allow students to express their knowledge and understanding of the subject matter or to present a personal opinion. The questions may be used to stimulate class discussion. Because answers to these questions may vary, determination of the answer's acceptability is left to the discretion of the course instructor.

1. How is PET/CT scanning accomplished? What value does this modality have in diagnosing the spread of cancer in the human body?

2. What are some of the problems that may be encountered in designing shielding for a PET/CT department?

3. During a radiation emergency situation, what role does a radiologic technologist in a health care facility fulfill?

4. When medical care is being provided to a patient contaminated with radiation either externally or internally, what protective measures should be taken by physicians and staff members coming in contact with the patient?

5. Describe a scenario that involves a radioactive dispersal device (dirty bomb). Include possible health and community consequences and the emergency response to the situation, with emphasis on radiation safety.

POST-TEST

The student should take this test after reading Chapter 13, finishing all accompanying textbook and workbook exercises, and completing any additional activities required by the course instructor. The student should complete the post-test with a score of 90% or higher before advancing to the next chapter. (Each of the following 20 questions or blanks is worth 5 points.) Score = _____ %

1. What U.S. government agency facilitates the development and enforcement of regulations controlling radiation in the environment and sets limits for radioactive contamination that assume that a 1-in-10,000 risk of causing a fatal cancer is unacceptable?

2. Define *radioactive dispersal device*.

_____

_____

3. How are therapeutic radioisotopes characterized?

_____

_____

4. ^{18}F has a physical half-life of:
   A. 110 seconds
   B. 110 minutes
   C. 110 hours
   D. 110 years

5. Isotopes are atoms that have the same number of protons in the nucleus but have different numbers of _____.

6. _____ dividing cells that are well oxygenated are very radiosensitive.

7. What is a neutrino?

_____

_____

8. After a dirty bomb explosion, how can externally contaminated individuals be decontaminated?

_____

_____

9. Of what radiation events does PET make use?

_____

10. A 1-in-10,000 probability of causing a fatal cancer corresponds to an effective dose of approximately _____ mSv (_____ mrem).

11. A radioactive tracer that is taken up or metabolized by cancerous cells and that also will reveal their locations through its positron emission decay and subsequent generation of oppositely traveling annihilation photons is _____.

12. Diagnostic techniques in nuclear medicine typically make use of _____ radioisotopes as radioactive tracers.

13. During an emergency, under what dose limit are individuals performing lifesaving activities allowed to work?

_____

14. Define the term *electron capture*.

_____

_____

15. In what do positron emitters result?

16. What radiation survey instrument is used by emergency personnel to monitor radioactive contamination?

17. What radioisotope is most often used in nuclear medicine diagnostic studies?

18. What do most hospitals have for handling emergency situations involving radioactive contamination?

19. A well-designed PET/CT facility is arranged so that no areas of full occupancy are adjacent to a _____ radiation source.

20. Fast-moving electrons are _____ radiation.

Answer Key

Chapter 1

Exercise 1: Crossword Puzzle

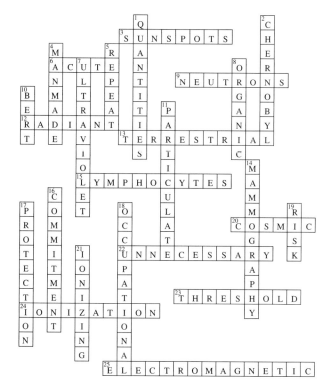

Exercise 2: Matching

1. P	6. A	11. I	16. J	21. L
2. X	7. H	12. E	17. O	22. S
3. F	8. Y	13. T	18. R	23. M
4. C	9. G	14. D	19. N	24. Q
5. K	10. B	15. W	20. U	25. V

Exercise 3: Multiple Choice

1. C	6. C	11. C	16. B	21. D
2. B	7. D	12. D	17. C	22. C
3. C	8. B	13. D	18. D	23. D
4. A	9. B	14. D	19. C	24. B
5. B	10. C	15. B	20. A	25. C

Exercise 4: True or False

1. T
2. T
3. T
4. F (No threshold exists.)
5. F (3 mSv/yr [approximately 300 mrem/yr])
6. T
7. F (They vary.)
8. F (EqD enables the calculation of EfD.)
9. F (They are continuously exposed.)
10. T
11. F (No atmospheric nuclear testing has occurred since 1980.)
12. F (They produce negligible radiation exposure.)
13. T
14. T
15. F (Alpha particles can be absorbed; they are very damaging to radiosensitive epithelial tissue.)
16. F (approximately 0.3 mSv [30 mrem]/yr)
17. T
18. T
19. F (A neutron has approximately the same mass as a proton.)
20. F (a classic example of organic damage)
21. T
22. F (Smokers exposed to high radon levels have a higher risk of lung cancer than do nonsmokers.)
23. F (Solar contribution to the cosmic ray background increases.)
24. T
25. T

Exercise 5: Fill in the Blank

1. radiation dose, dose rates
2. latent period
3. ETHOS Project
4. benefits, far outweigh, risk
5. energy, biologic effects
6. terrestrial
7. Cosmic
8. radionuclides
9. equivalent dose
10. x-ray machines, radiopharmaceuticals
11. safe operation
12. wave-particle duality
13. ALARA
14. BERT, comparison
15. radon, lung
16. radionuclides
17. greatest, lowest
18. 600, 60,000
19. 0.0116, 1.16
20. Thyroid
21. justify, responsibility
22. beneficial, destructive
23. 40, molten
24. higher
25. frequencies, wavelengths

Exercise 6: Labeling

A.

1. Glass envelope
2. Target (anode +)
3. High-speed electron stream
4. Filament (cathode −)
5. X-ray beam (electromagnetic waves)

B.

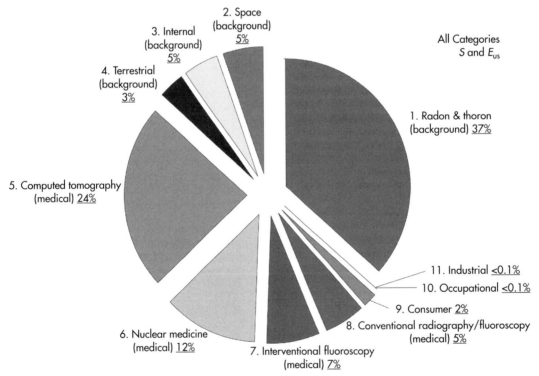

All Categories S and E_{us}

1. Radon & thoron (background) 37%
2. Space (background) 5%
3. Internal (background) 5%
4. Terrestrial (background) 3%
5. Computed tomography (medical) 24%
6. Nuclear medicine (medical) 12%
7. Interventional fluoroscopy (medical) 7%
8. Conventional radiography/fluoroscopy (medical) 5%
9. Consumer 2%
10. Occupational ≤0.1%
11. Industrial ≤0.1%

From National Council on Radiation Protection and Measurements (NCRP): *Ionizing radiation exposure of the population of the United States,* Report No. 160, Bethesda, Md, 2009, NRCP.

C.

Radiation Equivalent Dose and Subsequent Biologic Effects Resulting from Acute Whole Body Exposures*

Radiation Equivalent Dose (EqD)	Subsequent Biologic Effect
1. 0.25 Sv (25 rem)	Blood changes (e.g., measurable hematologic depression, decreases in the number of lymphocytes present in the circulating blood)
2. 1.5 Sv (150 rem)	Nausea, diarrhea
3. 2.0 Sv (200 rem)	Erythema (diffuse redness over an area of skin after irradiation)
4. 2.5 Sv (250 rem)	If dose is to gonads, temporary sterility
5. 3.0 Sv (300 rem)	50% chance of death; lethal dose for 50% of population over 30 days (LD 50/30)
6. 6.0 Sv (600 rem)	Death

Modified from *Radiologic health,* unit 4, slide 17, Denver, Multi-Media Publishing (slide program).
*Radiation exposures are delivered to the entire body over a time period of less than a few hours.

Exercise 7: Short Answer

1. Humans can safely control the use of radiant energy by using the knowledge of radiation hazards that has been gained over many years and by employing effective methods to limit or eliminate those hazards.
2. Radiologic technologists and radiologists can reduce radiation exposure to patients and to themselves by using protective devices whenever possible, by following established procedures, and by selecting technical exposure factors that significantly reduce radiation exposure.
3. Ionizing radiation produces damage while penetrating body tissue, primarily by ejecting electrons from the atoms composing the tissues.
4. The amount of energy transferred to electrons by ionizing radiation is the basis of the concept of radiation dose.
5. If excessive cellular damage occurs as a consequence of radiation exposure, the living organism exhibits genetic or somatic changes.
6. Cosmic rays are of extraterrestrial origin. They result from nuclear interactions that have taken place on the sun and other stars.
7. Potassium-40 (^{40}K); carbon-14 (^{14}C); hydrogen-3 (^{3}H; tritium); and strontium-90 (^{90}Sr).
8. The total annual equivalent dose from fallout cannot be estimated accurately because actual radiation measurements do not exist. The dose commitment may be estimated by using a series of approximations and simplistic models that are subject to considerable speculation.
9. When ionizing radiation is used for the welfare of the patient, the directly realized benefits of the exposure to this radiant energy must far outweigh any slight risk of induction of a radiogenic malignancy or genetic defect.
10. The patient dose for each x-ray procedure varies from one health care facility to another because of the large variety of radiologic equipment and the differences in imaging procedures and the technical skills of individual radiologists and radiographers.
11. Six consequences of ionization in human cells are (1) creation of unstable atoms; (2) production of free electrons; (3) production of low-energy x-ray photons; (4) creation of reactive free radicals capable of producing substances poisonous to the cell; (5) creation of new biologic molecules detrimental to the living cell; and (6) injury to the cell that may manifest itself as abnormal function or loss of function.
12. Nonionizing infrared and ultraviolet radiation actually produces the sensation of heat or the chemical changes that produce suntan and sunburn.
13. The millirem, a subunit of the rem, is equal to $^{1}/_{1000}$ of a rem.
14. Six sources of manmade (artificial) ionizing radiation are (1) consumer products containing radioactive material; (2) air travel; (3) nuclear fuel for generating power; (4) atmospheric fallout from nuclear weapons testing; (5) nuclear power plant accidents; and (6) medical radiation.
15. Using the background equivalent radiation time (BERT) method to compare the amount of radiation received with natural background radiation received over a given period has three advantages: (1) BERT does not imply radiation risk, but rather is simply a means of comparison; (2) BERT emphasizes that radiation is an innate part of our environment; and (3) an answer given in terms of BERT is easy for the patient to comprehend.
16. Thyroid cancer continues to be the main adverse health effect of the 1986 accident at the Chernobyl nuclear power plant.
17. Three ways of indicating the amount of radiation received by a patient are (1) entrance skin exposure (ESE); (2) bone marrow dose; and (3) gonadal dose.
18. The radiation quantity equivalent dose (EqD) enables the calculation of the effective dose (EfD).
19. Kinetic energy is energy of motion.
20. In terms of ability to penetrate biologic matter, alpha particles are less penetrating than beta particles. Because alpha particles lose energy quickly as they travel a short distance through biologic matter (e.g., into the superficial layers of the skin), they are considered virtually harmless as an external source of radiation.

Exercise 8: General Discussion or Opinion Questions

The questions in this exercise are intended to allow students to express their knowledge and understanding of the subject matter covered in this chapter. Because the answers may vary, determination of an answer's acceptability is left to the discretion of the instructor.

Post-Test

1. *Radiation protection* may be defined as effective measures used by radiation workers to safeguard patients, personnel, and the general public from unnecessary exposure to ionizing radiation.
2. As low as reasonably achievable (ALARA)
3. The referring physician

4. risk
5. An effective radiation safety program
6. Electrically charged particles
7. effective
8. The sievert (Sv) is the SI unit of measure, and the rem is the traditional unit of measure for the EqD and EfD.
9. B
10. D
11. The amount of radiation received by a patient
12. The electromagnetic spectrum
13. Natural sources of ionizing radiation
14. Background equivalent radiation time (BERT)
15. C
16. D
17. As an internal source of radiation
18. repeated
19. Thyroid cancer
20. Genetic damage

Chapter 2
Exercise 1: Crossword Puzzle

Exercise 2: Matching
1. G
2. O
3. K
4. P
5. D
6. M
7. J
8. C
9. Q
10. L
11. N
12. I
13. A
14. R
15. H
16. F
17. S
18. B
19. T
20. U
21. E
22. V
23. Y
24. X
25. W

Exercise 3: Multiple Choice
1. D
2. D
3. B
4. A
5. C
6. B
7. D
8. B
9. B
10. B
11. D
12. C
13. B
14. D
15. A
16. C
17. D
18. C
19. C
20. C
21. D
22. D
23. A
24. C
25. C

Exercise 4: True or False
1. T
2. F (direct transmission)
3. T
4. F (outer-shell electron)
5. T
6. F (They must be different.)
7. T
8. F (It is not.)
9. T
10. F (increase in absorbed dose)
11. T
12. F (secondary, or recoil, electron)
13. T
14. T
15. F (It can cause excitation or ionization until all its kinetic energy has been spent.)
16. F (decreasing the intensity of the primary photon beam)
17. F (Characteristic radiation is also emitted from the atom.)
18. F (The minimum energy required to produce an electron-positron pair is 1.022 MeV.)
19. F (The target in the x-ray tube is also known as the *anode*.)
20. T
21. T
22. T
23. F (The Z_{eff} of air is 7.6)
24. T
25. T

Exercise 5: Fill in the Blank
1. manmade
2. electrons, photons
3. electrical voltage
4. degrade
5. image
6. coherent (elastic, or unmodified)
7. forward, backward
8. Compton, photoelectric
9. Auger
10. absorption
11. electrons, positively
12. energy, energy
13. one third
14. intensity
15. Rayleigh, Thompson
16. darker
17. increase
18. antimatter
19. photoelectric, Compton
20. Coherent (classical, elastic, unmodified)
21. kVp
22. increases, decreases, increases
23. absorption
24. recoil
25. kinetic

Exercise 6: Labeling

A.

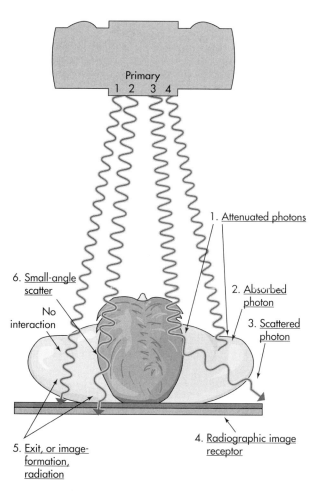

1. Attenuated photons
2. Absorbed photon
3. Scattered photon
4. Radiographic image receptor
5. Exit, or image-formation, radiation
6. Small-angle scatter

Primary − Exit = Attenuation

B.

1. Outer shell electron
2. Scattered photon of less energy
3. Compton scattered electron

C.

1. Inner shell electron
2. Photoelectron
3. Negatively charged photoelectron
4. Inner shell vacancy
5. Filled by outer shell electrons—causing radiation

Exercise 7: Short Answer

1. Five types of interactions between x-radiation and matter are possible: (1) coherent (classical, elastic, or unmodified) scattering; (2) Compton (incoherent, inelastic, or modified) scattering; (3) photoelectric absorption; (4) pair production; and (5) photodisintegration.

2. Because the level of energy (beam quality) and the number of x-ray photons are controlled by technique factors selected by the radiographer, the radiographer is actually responsible for the dose the patient receives during an imaging procedure. With a suitable understanding of these factors, radiographers can select appropriate techniques that can minimize the dose to the patient and produce optimal-quality images.

3. Absorption and the differences in the absorption properties of various body structures makes it possible to produce diagnostically useful images in which different anatomic structures can be perceived and distinguished.

4. Reducing the amount of tissue irradiated reduces the amount of fog produced by small-angle scatter. The radiographer can collimate the x-ray beam to reduce the amount of tissue irradiated.
5. The energy of the electrons inside a diagnostic x-ray tube is expressed in terms of the electrical voltage applied across the tube. In diagnostic radiology, this is expressed in thousands of volts, or kilovolts (kV). Because the voltage across the tube fluctuates, it usually is expressed in kilovolt peak (kVp).
6. The minimum energy required to produce an electron-positron pair is 1.022 MeV.
7. Positive contrast media consist of solutions containing elements having a higher atomic number than surrounding tissue (e.g., barium or iodine based) that are either ingested or injected into the tissues or structures to be visualized.
8. Three unstable nuclei used in positron emission tomography (PET) scanning are fluorine-18 (^{18}F), carbon-11 (^{11}C), and nitrogen-13 (^{13}N).
9. A photoelectron has kinetic energy equal to the energy of the incident photon less the binding energy of the electron shell.
10. Scattered radiation may contribute to degradation of the radiographic image by creating an additional, unwanted density, radiographic fog.
11. The two methods most often used to limit the effects of indirectly transmitted x-ray photons are air gaps and radiographic grids.
12. During the process of coherent scattering, because the wavelengths of both incident and scattered waves are the same, no net energy is absorbed by the atom.
13. Mass density is the quantity of matter per unit volume. It generally is specified in units of kilograms per cubic meter (kg/m^3) or grams per cubic centimeter (g/cc).
14. Radiographic contrast is the difference in density level between the radiographic images of objects in an image.
15. Annihilation radiation is used in PET.

Exercise 8: General Discussion or Opinion Questions

The questions in this exercise are intended to allow students to express their knowledge and understanding of the subject matter covered in this chapter. Because the answers may vary, determination of an answer's acceptability is left to the discretion of the instructor.

Post-Test

1. photoelectric
2. Attenuation is any process decreasing the intensity of the primary photon beam that was directed toward a destination.
3. minimizes
4. personnel
5. partially
6. peak kilovoltage (kVp)
7. random
8. photodisintegration
9. photoelectric absorption
10. C
11. A
12. B
13. A
14. D
15. A
16. 13.8
17. absorbed dose
18. contrast
19. all-directional
20. The term *fluorescent yield* refers to the number of x-rays emitted per inner-shell vacancy.

Chapter 3

Exercise 1: Crossword Puzzle

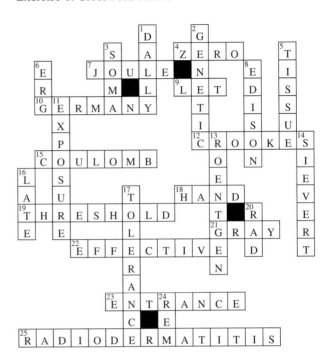

Exercise 2: Matching
1. J
2. D
3. C
4. G
5. E
6. L
7. O
8. B
9. Y
10. M
11. S
12. N
13. H
14. T
15. W
16. A
17. K
18. P
19. F
20. X
21. I
22. U
23. Q
24. R
25. V

Exercise 3: Multiple Choice
1. C
2. A
3. D
4. C
5. D
6. D
7. C
8. C
9. A
10. D
11. B
12. D
13. C
14. D
15. A
16. B
17. A
18. C
19. D
20. C
21. D
22. B
23. D
24. D
25. A

Exercise 4: True or False
1. T
2. F (The paper was coated with barium platinocyanide.)
3. T
4. T
5. F (the maximum permissible dose [MPD])
6. F (revised by the International Commission on Radiological Protection [ICRP], studies of the atomic bomb survivors)
7. T
8. F (Louis Harold Gray)
9. T
10. F (sievert and rem)
11. F (used for the radiation quantity, exposure, in air only)
12. T
13. T
14. F (number of electron-ion pairs also increases)
15. T
16. F (Skin erythema dose was a crude and inaccurate means of measuring radiation exposure because the amount of radiation required to produce erythema varies from person to person.)
17. T

18. T
19. F (The higher the atomic number of a material, the more x-ray energy it absorbs.)
20. T
21. F (It may be determined and expressed in sieverts or in rem.)
22. T
23. F (The gray [Gy] or rad is used for the absorbed dose [D] measurement.)
24. T
25. T

Exercise 5: Fill in the Blank

1. Wilhelm Conrad Roentgen
2. cancerous
3. erythema
4. exposure
5. organs, organ systems
6. absorbed dose
7. coulomb
8. biologic effect
9. sieverts, rem
10. risk, entire
11. radiation equivalent man
12. nonhazardous
13. different
14. quantities, units
15. workable
16. roentgen
17. 0.2, 0.1
18. roentgen
19. safety
20. SI
21. Louis Harold Gray
22. Rolf Maximilian Sievert
23. measure
24. ionization (charge)
25. temperature, pressure, humidity

Exercise 6: Labeling

A.

B.

Radiation Weighting Factors for Different Types and Energies of Ionizing Radiation

Radiation Type and Energy Range	Radiation Weighting Factor (W_R)
X-ray and gamma ray photons, electrons (every energy)	1. 1
Neutrons, energy <10 keV	2. 5
10 to 100 keV	3. 10
>100 keV to 2 MeV	4. 20
>2 to 20 MeV	5. 10
>20 MeV	6. 5
Protons	7. 2
Alpha particles	8. 20

Data adapted from International Commission on Radiological Protection (ICRP): *Recommendations,* ICRP Publication No. 60, New York, 1991, Pergamon Press.

C.

Summary of Radiation Quantities and Units

Type of Radiation	Quantity	SI	Traditional Unit	Measuring Medium	Radiation Effect Measured
X-radiation or gamma	1. Exposure (X)	Coulomb per kilogram (C/kg)	Roentgen (R)	Air	Ionization of air radiation
All ionizing radiations	2. Absorbed dose (D)	Gray (Gy)	Rad	Any object	Amount of energy per unit mass absorbed by object
All ionizing radiations	3. Equivalent dose (EqD)	Sievert (Sv)	Rem	Body tissue	Biologic effects
All ionizing radiations	4. Effective dose (Efd)	Sievert (Sv)	Rem	Body tissue	Biologic a effects

Exercise 7: Short Answer

1. Thomas A. Edison discontinued his x-ray research because of the severe injuries and death of his friend, Clarence Dally, which were attributed to radiation-induced cancer.
2. Skin erythema dose was the unit used for measuring radiation exposure from 1900 to 1930.
3. Short-term (early or acute) somatic effects of ionizing radiation are effects that appear within minutes, hours, days, or weeks of the time of radiation exposure. Long-term, or late, somatic effects appear months or years after exposure to ionizing radiation.
4. Tolerance dose is a radiation dose to which occupationally exposed persons could be continuously subjected without any apparent harmful acute effects, such as erythema of the skin.
5. Maximum permissible dose (or MPD) replaced tolerance dose for radiation protection purposes in the 1950s.
6. In the late 1970s, dose limits were calculated and established to ensure that the risk from radiation exposure acquired while on the job did not exceed risks encountered in "safe" occupations, such as clerical work in which the risk is approximately 10^{-4} per year.
7. The Bragg-Gray theory relates the ionization produced in a small cavity within an irradiated medium or object to the energy absorbed in that medium as a result of its radiation exposure. With the use of appropriate correction factors, the theory essentially links the determination of the absorbed radiation dose in a medium to a relatively simple measurement of ionization charge. The Bragg-Gray theory is the most important theory in all of radiation dosimetry.
8. When the human body is exposed to ionizing radiation, absorbed energy is responsible for any biologic damage to the tissues resulting from this exposure.
9. For precise measurement of radiation exposure in radiography, the total amount of ionization (charge) an x-ray beam produces in a known mass of air must be obtained. This type of direct measurement is accomplished in an accredited calibration laboratory using a standard or free air ionization chamber.
10. The radiation weighting factors are selected by national and international scientific advisory bodies (NCRP, ICRP) and are based on quality factors and linear energy transfer.
11. If absorbed dose is stated in rad, the equivalent number of gray may be determined by dividing the rad value by 100.
12. If absorbed dose is stated in gray, the number of rad may be determined by multiplying the gray value by 100.
13. Coulomb per kilogram (C/kg) or roentgen (R) is used for x-ray equipment calibration because x-ray output is measured directly with an ionization chamber.
14. If the radiation exposure is given in R, it can be converted to C/kg by multiplying the number of roentgens by 2.58×10^{-4}.
15. If the radiation exposure is given in C/kg, it can be converted to R by dividing by 2.58×10^{-4}.

Exercise 8: General Discussion or Opinion Questions

The questions in this exercise are intended to allow students to express their knowledge and understanding of the subject matter covered in this chapter. Because the answers may vary, determination of an answer's acceptability is left to the discretion of the instructor.

Exercise 9: Calculation Problems

A.
1. 8000 rad = 8000 ÷ 100 rad per Gy = 80 Gy
2. 8 rad = 8 ÷ 100 rad per Gy = 0.08 Gy
3. 450 rad = 450 ÷ 100 rad per Gy = 4.5 Gy
4. 4.5 rad = 4.5 ÷ 100 rad per Gy = 0.045 Gy
5. 375 rad = 375 ÷ 100 rad per Gy = 3.75 Gy
6. 7 Gy = 7 × 100 rad per Gy = 700 rad
7. 25 Gy = 25 × 100 rad per Gy = 2500 rad
8. 0.4 Gy = 0.4 × 100 rad per Gy = 40 rad
9. 0.087 Gy = 0.087 × 100 rad per Gy = 8.7 rad
10. 0.96 Gy = 0.96 × 100 rad per Gy = 96 rad

B.

1.

Radiation Type	D	×	WR	=	EqD
X-radiation	0.6 Gy	×	1	=	0.6 Sv
Fast neutrons	0.25 Gy	×	20	=	5 Sv
Alpha particles	0.4 Gy	×	20	=	8 Sv
			Total EqD	=	13.6 Sv

2.

Radiation Type	D	×	W_R	=	EqD
X-radiation	0.3 Gy	×	1	=	0.3 Sv
Fast neutrons	0.28 Gy	×	20	=	5.6 Sv
Gamma rays	0.8 Gy	×	1	=	0.8 Sv
Protons	0.9 Gy	×	2	=	1.8 Sv
Alpha particles	0.4 Gy	×	20	=	8 Sv
			Total EqD	=	16.5 Sv

3.

Radiation Type	D	×	W_R	=	EqD
X-radiation	7 rad	×	1	=	7 rem
Fast neutrons	2 rad	×	20	=	40 rem
Alpha particles	5 rad	×	20	=	100 rem
			Total EqD	=	147 rem

4.

Radiation Type	D	×	W_R	=	EqD
X-radiation	3 rad	×	1	=	3 rem
Fast neutrons	0.35 rad	×	20	=	7 rem
Gamma rays	6 rad	×	1	=	6 rem
Protons	2.5 rad	×	2	=	5 rem
Alpha particles	8 rad	×	20	=	160 rem
			Total EqD	=	181 rem

5.

Radiation Type	D	×	W_R	=	EqD
X-radiation	0.6 Gy	×	1	=	0.6 Sv
Fast neutrons, energy<10 keV	0.2 Gy	×	5	=	1 Sv
Gamma rays	4 Gy	×	1	=	4 Sv
Protons	0.8 Gy	×	2	=	1.6 Sv
Alpha particles	6 Gy	×	20	=	120 Sv
			Total EqD	=	127.2 Sv

C.

	D	×	W_R	×	W_T	=	EfD
1.	0.5 Gy	×	20	×	0.05	=	0.5 Sv
2.	0.4 Gy	×	1	×	0.2	=	0.08 Sv
3.	6 rad	×	20	×	0.12	=	14.4 rem
4.	25 rad	×	1	×	0.05	=	1.25 rem
5.	0.9 Gy	×	1	×	0.12	=	0.108 Sv

D.

	Number Exposed	×	Average EfD (Sv)	=	ColEfD
1.	400	×	0.2	=	80 person-sievert (80 × 100 = 8000 man-rem)
2.	300	×	0.17	=	51 person-sievert (51 × 100 = 5100 man-rem)
3.	250	×	0.24	=	60 person-sievert (60 × 100 = 6000 man-rem)
4.	1000	×	0.1	=	100 person-sievert (100 × 100 = 10,000 man-rem)
5.	100	×	0.3	=	30 person-sievert (30 × 100 = 3000 man-rem)

Post-Test

1. Number exposed × Average EfD = ColEfD
   400 × 0.2 Sv = 80 person-sievert (80 × 100 = 8000 man-rem)
2. Effective dose (EfD)
3. Linear energy transfer (LET)
4. The radiation quantity exposure (X) is expressed in coulombs per kilogram (C/kg) in the SI system and in roentgens (R) in the traditional system.
5. Leukemia
6. Wilhelm Conrad Roentgen
7.

Radiation Type	D	×	W_R	=	EqD
X-radiation	5 Gy	×	1	=	5 Sv
Fast neutrons	0.3 Gy	×	20	=	1.5 Sv
Alpha particles	0.7 Gy	×	20	=	14 Sv
				Total EqD	= 20.5 Sv

8. $D × W_R × W_T = EfD$
   $5\,Gy × 1 × 0.12 = 0.6\,Sv$
9. 800
10. $EqD = D × W_R$
11. A
12. C
13. Skin erythema
14. coulomb (c)
15. D
16. 10
17. centigray (cGy)
18. cancerous
19. Radiation exposure received by radiation workers in the course of exercising their professional responsibilities
20. The energy deposited in biologic tissue by ionizing radiation

Chapter 4

Exercise 1: Crossword Puzzle

(Crossword puzzle with answers including: PERSONNEL, LIGHTWEIGHT, ELECTROMETER, THERMOLUMINESCENT, LUMINESCENCE, TWO, COPPER, CALIBRATION, IMMEDIATE, FUZZY, GESTATION, EXTREMITY, DARKEN)

Exercise 2: Matching

1. K	6. N	11. Y	16. Q	21. J
2. M	7. B	12. W	17. D	22. S
3. L	8. O	13. R	18. G	23. X
4. C	9. A	14. P	19. E	24. V
5. H	10. I	15. U	20. F	25. T

Exercise 3: Multiple Choice

1. D	6. B	11. A	16. A	21. A
2. B	7. C	12. D	17. C	22. C
3. A	8. C	13. D	18. D	23. A
4. C	9. B	14. D	19. A	24. D
5. C	10. A	15. A	20. A	25. B

Exercise 4: True or False

1. F (They do not protect the wearer from ionizing radiation.)
2. T
3. T
4. F (It is a factor; personnel dosimeters selected for use must be cost effective.)
5. F (should be made of plastic of a low atomic number)
6. F (Exposure time is too short to allow the meter to respond.)
7. T
8. T
9. F (not equally sensitive in the detection of ionizing radiation)
10. T
11. F (usually for 1 month)
12. T
13. T
14. F (made out of aluminum, copper, and tin)
15. T
16. T
17. F (An optically stimulated luminescence [OSL] dosimeter can be worn up to 1 year; it commonly is worn for 2 months.)
18. T
19. T
20. F (A thermoluminescent dosimeter [TLD] can be read only once because the reading destroys the stored information.)
21. T
22. T
23. T
24. T
25. T

Exercise 5: Fill in the Blank

1. thyroid, eyes
2. annually
3. ionization, optically stimulated, thermoluminescent
4. inexpensive
5. sharply defined
6. radiation-free
7. equivalent
8. trigger
9. charged, zero
10. Medical physicists. electrometers
11. sensitive
12. lost, contamination
13. radiation output
14. occupational

15. laser light
16. second, gestation
17. deep, shallow
18. reused, cost-effective
19. Control
20. usage, placement
21. densitometer
22. worn
23. legal
24. 5, 40
25. plastic

Exercise 6: Labeling

A. Pocket ionization chamber (pocket dosimeter)

1. Quartz fiber indicator
2. Scale of built-in electrometer (of self-reading pocket dosimeter)

Exercise 7: Short Answer

1. By detecting and measuring the quantity of ionizing radiation to which the dosimeter has been exposed over a period of time.
2. Like traditional film badge monitors, OSL dosimeters must be shipped to the monitoring company for reading and exposure determination. This task takes time.
3. An extremity dosimeter measures the approximate equivalent dose to the hands of the wearer of the dosimeter.
4. The badge cover of an extremity monitor contains information such as the account number, participant's name and number, wear date, indication of hand (right or left), size, and reference number of the TLD ring dosimeter. All of this is laser etched to ensure permanent identification.
5. Optical density is the intensity of light transmitted through a given area of the dosimetry film.
6. Three radiation survey instruments used for area monitoring are the ionization chamber–type survey meter (cutie pie), the proportional counter, and the Geiger-Müller (GM) detector.
7. Proportional counters are generally used in a laboratory to detect alpha and beta radiation and small amounts of other types of low-level radioactive contamination.
8. Some disadvantages of the TLD are (1) the initial high cost; (2) the fact that it can be read only once because the readout process destroys the stored information; and (3) the fact that calibrated dosimeters must be used with TLDs.
9. The OSL dosimeter contains an aluminum oxide (Al_2O_3) detector (thin layer).
10. Radiation dosimetry film is sensitive to doses ranging from as low as 0.1 mSv (10 mrem) to as high as 5000 mSv (500 rem).
11. Because a GM tube tends to lose its calibration over time, it has a "check source" to verify its constancy daily.
12. When a protective lead apron is used during fluoroscopy or special procedures, the personnel dosimeter should be worn outside the apron at collar level on the anterior surface of the body because the unprotected head, neck, and lenses of the eyes receive 10 to 20 times more exposure than the protected body trunk. When the personnel dosimeter is located at collar level, it also provides a reading of the approximate equivalent dose to the thyroid gland and eyes of the occupationally exposed person.
13. The cumulative columns provide a continuous audit of actual absorbed radiation equivalent dose.
14. When the letter *M* appears under the current monitoring period or in the cumulative columns of a personnel monitoring report, it signifies that an equivalent dose below the minimum measurable radiation quantity was recorded during that time.
15. When changing employment, a radiation worker must convey the data pertinent to the accumulated permanent equivalent dose to the new employer so that this information can be placed on file.

Exercise 8: General Discussion or Opinion Questions

The questions in this exercise are intended to allow students to express their knowledge and understanding of the subject matter covered in this chapter. Because the answers may vary, determination of an answer's acceptability is left to the discretion of the instructor.

Post-Test

1. effective
2. An OSL dosimeter is a device for monitoring personnel exposure. It contains an aluminum oxide detector. The dosimeter is read out by using laser light at selected frequencies. When such laser light is incident on the sensing material, it becomes luminescent in proportion to the amount of radiation exposure received.
3. The working habits and working conditions of diagnostic imaging personnel can be assessed over a designated period of time through the use of the personnel dosimeter.
4. results
5. attached to the clothing on the front of the body at collar level
6. A
7. D
8. In a health care facility, a radiographer's deep, eye, and shallow occupational exposure as measured by an exposed monitor may be found on the personnel monitoring report.
9. A GM detector
10. zero (0)
11. abdomen
12. The data pertinent to the accumulated permanent equivalent dose so that it may be placed on file with the new employer
13. presence, absence, intensity, intensity rates
14. employment
15. Radiation workers are required to wear personnel monitoring devices whenever they are likely to risk receiving 10% or more of the annual EfD limit of 50 mSv (5 rem) in any one year as a consequence of their work-related activities.
16. primary
17. the radiation safety officer (RSO)
18. 2
19. ionization chambers
20. pregnant

Chapter 5

Exercise 1: Crossword Puzzle

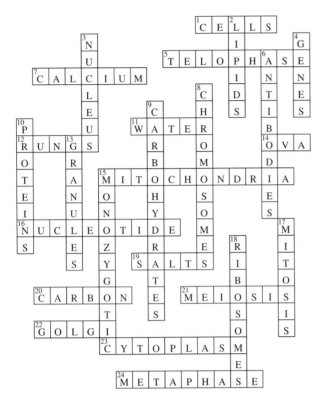

Exercise 2: Matching

1. D	6. C	11. E	16. J	21. Y
2. M	7. N	12. R	17. U	22. X
3. L	8. A	13. H	18. I	23. V
4. K	9. P	14. T	19. B	24. S
5. F	10. G	15. O	20. W	25. Q

Exercise 3: Multiple Choice

1. C	6. B	11. A	16. B	21. D
2. B	7. D	12. C	17. A	22. C
3. C	8. B	13. B	18. D	23. B
4. B	9. C	14. B	19. D	24. B
5. D	10. B	15. C	20. C	25. C

Exercise 4: True or False

1. T
2. F (80% to 85%)
3. T
4. F (The body's primary defense mechanism against infection and disease is antibodies.)
5. T
6. F (hydrogen bonds)
7. T
8. T
9. F (occur in the cytoplasm)
10. T
11. T
12. T
13. F (It is frail, semipermeable, and flexible.)
14. T
15. T
16. T
17. F (during metaphase)
18. T
19. T
20. F (Glucose is the primary energy source.)
21. T
22. F (Cells are essential for life.)
23. T
24. F (Proteins contain the most carbon.)
25. F (Carbohydrates are most abundant in the liver and in muscle tissue.)

Exercise 5: Fill in the Blank

1. cell
2. homeostasis
3. 24
4. amino acids
5. repair enzymes
6. hormones
7. liver, muscle
8. DNA
9. osmotic
10. fraternal
11. DNA
12. high
13. fluid
14. metabolism
15. metabolism
16. Ribosomes
17. catalytic, repair
18. macromolecules
19. nucleus
20. endoplasmic reticulum
21. replication
22. lysosomes
23. oxidative
24. salts
25. electrolytes

Exercise 6: Labeling

A.

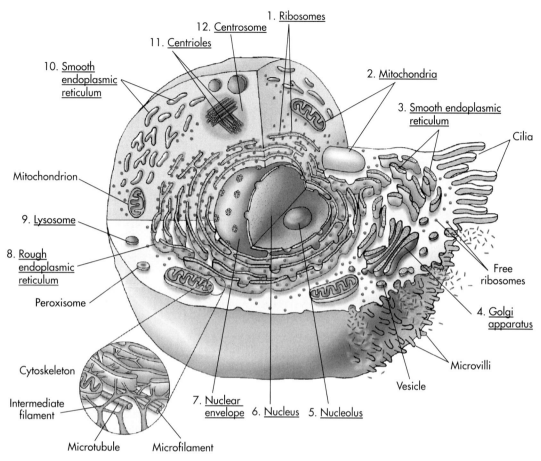

From Thibodeau A: *Anatomy and physiology,* ed 5, St Louis, 2003, Mosby.

B.

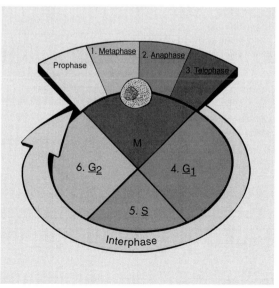

From Bushong SC: *Radiologic science for technologists: physics, biology, and protection,* ed 9, St Louis, 2008, Elsevier.

C.

Summary of Cell Components

Title	Site	Activity
1. Cell membrane	Cytoplasm	Functions as a barricade to protect cellular contents from their environment and controls the passage of water and other materials into and out of the cell; performs many additional functions such as elimination of wastes and refining of material for energy through breakdown of the materials
2. Endoplasmic reticulum	Cytoplasm	Enables the cell to communicate with the extracellular environment and transfers food from one part of the cell to another
3. Golgi apparatus	Cytoplasm	Unites large carbohydrate molecules and combines them with proteins to form glycoproteins and transports enzymes and hormones through the cell membrane so that they can exit the cell, enter the bloodstream, and be carried to areas of the body in which they are required
4. Mitochondria	Cytoplasm	Produce energy for cellular activity by breaking down nutrients through a process of oxidation
5. Lysosomes	Cytoplasm	Dispose of large particles such as bacteria and food as well as smaller particles; also contain hydrolytic enzymes that can break down and digest proteins, certain carbohydrates, and the cell itself if the lysosome's surrounding membrane breaks
6. Ribosomes	Cytoplasm	Manufacture the various proteins that cells require
7. Centrosomes	Cytoplasm	Believed to play some part in the formation of the mitotic spindle during cell division
8. DNA	Nucleus	Contains the genetic material, controls cell division and multiplication and also biochemical reactions that occur within the living cell
9. Nucleolus	Nucleus	Holds a large amount of RNA

Exercise 7: Short Answer

1. To ensure efficient cell operation, the body must provide food as a source of raw material for the release of energy, supply oxygen to help break down the food, and have enough water to transport inorganic substances such as calcium and sodium into and out of the cell.
2. Metabolism involves the reception and processing of food and oxygen and the elimination of waste products. It basically consists of chemical reactions in the body that modify food for cellular use. Metabolism enables the cell to perform the vital functions of synthesizing proteins and producing energy.
3. Proteins are formed when amino acids combine into long, chain-like molecular complexes. In these complexes a chemical link, called a *peptide bond,* connects each amino acid. Protein production, or *protein synthesis,* involves 22 different amino acids. The order of arrangement of these amino acids determines the precise function of each protein molecule.
4. Enzymatic proteins function as *organic catalysts,* agents that affect the rate of speed of chemical reactions without being altered themselves. Enzymatic proteins control the cell's various physiologic activities. Enzymes cause an increase in cellular activity, which in turn causes biochemical reactions to occur more rapidly to meet the needs of the cell. Hence, proper cell functioning depends on enzymes.
5. Lipids are fats or fatlike substances that are present in all body tissue. They perform many functions for the body; for example, they (1) act as reservoirs for long-term storage of energy; (2) insulate and guard the body against the environment; (3) support and protect organs such as the eyes and kidneys; (4) provide essential substances for growth and development; (5) lubricate the joints; and (6) assist in the digestive process.
6. Ribosomes function as protein factories for the cell; they manufacture (synthesize) the various proteins that cells require using the blueprints provided by messenger ribonucleic acid (mRNA).
7. Inside the cell, water is indispensable for metabolic activity because it is the medium in which the chemical reactions that are the bases of these activities occur. It also acts as a solvent, keeping compounds dissolved so that they can more easily interact and their concentration can be regulated. Outside the cell, water functions as a transport vehicle for minerals the cell uses or eliminates. In addition, water is responsible for maintaining a constant body core temperature of 98.6° F (37° C) and serving to lubricate both the digestive system and the skeletal articulations (joints). Organs such as the brain and lungs are also protected by a cushion of water.
8. The nucleus controls cell division and multiplication and the biochemical reactions that occur within the cell. By directing protein synthesis, the nucleus plays an essential role in active transport, metabolism, growth, and heredity.
9. Four distinct phases of the cellular life cycle are identifiable: M (mitosis phase), G_1 (pre–DNA synthesis phase), S (synthesis phase), and G_2 (post–DNA synthesis phase).
10. Carbohydrates are referred to as *saccharides.* A monosaccharide is a simple sugar molecule (e.g., glucose). A disaccharide is made up of two units of a simple sugar linked together (e.g., sucrose [cane sugar] and lactose). A *polysaccharide* is composed of several or many molecules of a simple sugar. Plant starches and animal glycogen are the two most important polysaccharides. Through the process of metabolism, the body breaks these down into simpler sugars for energy.
11. The four major classes of organic compounds in the human body are proteins, carbohydrates, lipids (fats), and nucleic acids.
12. Deoxyribonucleic acid (DNA) is a type of nucleic acid that carries the genetic information necessary for cell replication and regulates all cellular activity to direct protein synthesis.
13. Structural proteins, such as those found in muscle, provide the body with its shape and form and are a source of heat and energy.

14. In the nucleus of a living cell two nuclear components, DNA and protein, are arranged in long threads called *chromatin*. When a cell divides, this genetic-containing material contracts into tiny rod-shaped bodies called *chromosomes* that carry genes within their DNA.
15. Hormones are chemical secretions manufactured by various endocrine glands and carried by the bloodstream to influence the activities of other parts of the body. Hormones produced by the thyroid gland located in the neck control metabolism throughout the body. Hormones also regulate functions such as growth and development.

Exercise 8: General Discussion or Opinion Questions

The questions in this exercise are intended to allow students to express their knowledge and understanding of the subject matter covered in this chapter. Because the answers may vary, determination of an answer's acceptability is left to the discretion of the instructor.

Post-Test

1. matter
2. organic
3. repair enzymes
4. nitrogenous
5. water
6. The DNA macromolecule is composed of two long sugar-phosphate chains that twist around each other in a double-helix configuration. These chains are linked by pairs of nitrogenous organic bases at the sugar molecules of the chains. This forms a tightly coiled structure resembling a twisted ladder or spiral staircase. The sugar-phosphate compounds are the side rails, and the pairs of nitrogenous bases, which consist of complementary chemicals, are the steps, or rungs, of the DNA ladderlike structure. Hydrogen bonds attach the bases to each other, joining the two side rails of the DNA ladder.
7. mapping
8. C
9. C
10. During metaphase
11. Ribosomes synthesize the various proteins that cells require.
12. Approximately 30,000
13. The affected cells will function abnormally or die.
14. 22
15. A nucleotide
16. DNA
17. Cytoplasm
18. Interphase
19. Lipids
20. The cell membrane encases and surrounds the cell, functions as a barricade to protect cellular contents from the outside environment, and controls the passage of water and other materials into and out of the cell.

Chapter 6

Exercise 1: Crossword Puzzle

Exercise 2: Matching

1. N
2. O
3. H
4. D
5. E
6. L
7. A
8. K
9. I
10. F
11. B
12. G
13. M
14. J
15. C
16. Y
17. P
18. W
19. R
20. V
21. S
22. Q
23. X
24. U
25. T

Exercise 3: Multiple Choice

1. B
2. B
3. A
4. D
5. A
6. D
7. D
8. C
9. D
10. A
11. C
12. A
13. A
14. A
15. B
16. B
17. C
18. A
19. A
20. C

Exercise 4: True or False

1. F (can be damaged by radiation)
2. T
3. F (vary among the different types of ionizing radiation)
4. T
5. F (high-LET radiation)
6. F (are basically unstable)
7. T
8. F (contains large numbers of immature, unspecialized cells and is therefore radiosensitive)
9. T
10. T
11. F (deoxyribonucleic acid [DNA])
12. T
13. F (can adversely affect cell division)
14. T
15. T
16. T
17. F (The presence of free radicals dramatically increases the amount of biologic damage produced.)
18. F (X-ray photons may interact with and ionize water molecules in the human body.)
19. T
20. T
21. F (different types of cells and tissues, which vary in their degree of radiosensitivity)
22. F (In radiotherapy the presence of oxygen plays a significant role in radiosensitivity.)

23. F (the less sensitive it is to radiation)
24. T
25. T

Exercise 5: Fill in the Blank
1. cellular
2. energy
3. sublethal
4. mass, charge
5. internal
6. permanent
7. hydroxyl
8. gene
9. radiosensitivity
10. ionizing radiation
11. infection
12. platelets
13. granulocytes
14. decrease
15. mitosis
16. radiosensitive
17. radiosensitive
18. microcephaly (small head circumference), mental retardation
19. insensitive
20. radiosensitive
21. dies, restored
22. 2, 200
23. 5, 6, 500, 600
24. immature, susceptible
25. 0.25, 25

Exercise 6: Labeling
A.

B.

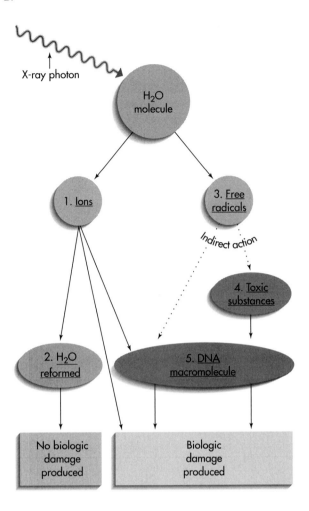

C. **Examples of Radiosensitive and Radioinsensitive Cells**

Radiosensitive Cells	Radioinsensitive Cells
1. Basal cells of the skin	4. Brain cells
2. Intestinal crypt cells	5. Muscle cells
3. Reproductive (germ) cells	6. Nerve cells

Exercise 7: Short Answer
1. High-energy charged particles (e.g., alpha and beta particles and protons) ionize atoms by interacting electromagnetically with orbital electrons. For example, an alpha particle that carries an electrical charge of plus two strongly attracts the negatively charged electron as it passes by.
2. Characteristics that vary (e.g., charge, mass, and energy) among the different types of radiations determine the extent to which different radiation modalities transfer energy into biologic tissue.
3. LET generally is described in units of kiloelectron volts (keV) per micron (1 micron [μm] = 10^{-6} m).
4. Repair enzymes usually can reverse the cellular damage caused by low-LET radiation because low-LET radiation generally causes sublethal damage to DNA.

5. Free radicals are solitary atoms or most often a combination of atoms that behave as extremely reactive single entities as a result of the presence of unpaired electrons.
6. All cells in the body other than female and male germ cells are classified as somatic cells.
7. Oxygen enhances the effects of ionizing radiation on biologic tissue by increasing tissue radiosensitivity. If oxygen is present when a tissue is irradiated, more free radicals are formed in the tissue; this increases the potential for indirect damage from radiation.
8. Damage to the cell's nucleus from ionizing radiation reveals itself in one of the following ways: instant death; reproductive death; apoptosis, or programmed cell death (interphase death); mitotic, or genetic, death; mitotic delay; interference with function; and chromosome breakage.
9. With *direct action,* biologic damage occurs as a result of ionization of atoms on master, or key, molecules (DNA), which can cause these molecules to become inactive or functionally altered. *Indirect action* refers to the effects produced by reactive free radicals that are created by the interaction of radiation with water (H_2O) molecules. These unstable, highly reactive agents have the potential to substantially disrupt master molecules, resulting in cell death.
10. If the nucleus in an adult nerve cell is destroyed by exposure to ionizing radiation, the cell dies and is never restored.
11. Even small doses of ionizing radiation (e.g., as low as 0.1 Gy [10 rad]) may cause menstrual irregularities, such as delay or suppression of menstruation.
12. Ionizing radiation interacts randomly with matter. Consequently, exposure to radiation produces a variety of structural changes in biologic tissue. Seven of these possible changes are (1) a single-strand break in one chromosome; (2) a single-strand break in one chromatid; (3) a single-strand break in separate chromosomes; (4) a strand break in separate chromatids; (5) more than one break in the same chromosome; (6) more than one break in the same chromatid; and (7) chromosome stickiness, or clumping.
13. Radiation damage is observed on three levels: molecular, cellular, and organic.
14. Ionizing radiation causes complete chromosome breakage when two direct hits occur in the same rung of a DNA macromolecule.
15. In 1906 two French scientists, J. Bergonié and L. Tribondeau, observed the effects of ionizing radiation on testicular germ cells of rabbits they had exposed to x-rays. They established that radiosensitivity was a function of the metabolic state of the cell receiving the exposure. Their findings eventually became known as the Law of Bergonié and Tribondeau, which states that the radiosensitivity of cells is directly proportional to their reproductive activity and inversely proportional to their degree of differentiation.

Exercise 8: General Discussion or Opinion Questions

The questions in this exercise are intended to allow students to express their knowledge and understanding of the subject matter covered in this chapter. Because the answers may vary, determination of an answer's acceptability is left to the discretion of the instructor.

Post-Test

1. The following formula is used:
   $$\frac{\text{Dose in Gy from 250 kVp x-rays (reference radiation)}}{\text{Dose in Gy of test radiation}} = \text{Relative biologic effectiveness (RBE)}$$
   $21 \div 7 = 3$
   RBE = 3
2. water
3. apoptosis
4. LET is the amount of energy transferred on average by incident radiation to an object per unit length of track during its passage through the object. It is described in units of keV/μm.
5. Oxygen enhancement ratio (OER)
6. direct
7. C
8. D
9. target
10. indirect
11. Lymphocytes
12. Law of Bergonié and Tribondeau
13. mutations
14. A cell survival curve is used to display the radiosensitivity of a particular type of cell, which helps determine the types of cancer cells that will respond to radiation therapy.
15. bond
16. a measurable hematologic depression
17. repopulate
18. blood count
19. mental retardation
20. Ionizing radiation causes complete chromosome breakage when two direct hits occur in the same rung of the DNA macromolecule.

Chapter 7

Exercise 1: Crossword Puzzle

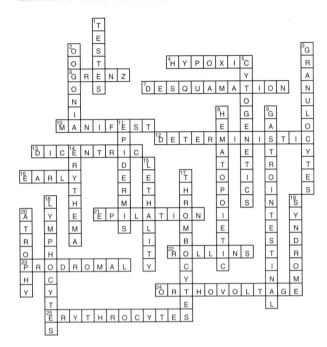

Exercise 2: Matching

1. O	6. N	11. Y	16. F	21. U
2. E	7. D	12. H	17. Q	22. W
3. M	8. G	13. X	18. C	23. S
4. K	9. J	14. B	19. V	24. R
5. A	10. I	15. P	20. L	25. T

Exercise 3: Multiple Choice

1. A	6. D	11. C	16. D	21. D
2. A	7. C	12. C	17. C	22. B
3. C	8. D	13. D	18. C	23. B
4. D	9. D	14. D	19. D	24. A
5. D	10. A	15. D	20. A	25. C

Exercise 4: True or False

1. F (They do not.)
2. F (The risk increases.)
3. F (metaphase)
4. T
5. T
6. F (decrease)
7. F (3 to 4 Gy [300 to 400 rad])
8. T
9. T
10. F (short period of time)
11. F (when a large dose of densely ionizing [high-LET] radiation is delivered to a large or radiosensitive area of the body)
12. F (high-LET radiation exposure)
13. T
14. F (a decrease)
15. T
16. F (Whole-body equivalent doses greater than 12 Gy [1200 rad] are considered fatal.)
17. T
18. T
19. F (during metaphase)
20. T
21. T
22. F (LD 50/60 may be more accurate.)
23. T
24. F (all layers of the skin and accessory organs)
25. T

Exercise 5: Fill in the Blank

1. substantial dose
2. 1, 100
3. radiation sickness
4. early, late
5. platelets
6. biologic criteria
7. death
8. repair, repopulation
9. functional
10. high
11. William Herbert Rollins
12. 2, 200
13. 10, 20
14. radiosensitive
15. menstruation
16. atrophy
17. chromosomal abnormalities
18. 0.25 (25)
19. anemia
20. indirect action
21. photograph, photomicrograph
22. direct action
23. ionizing radiation
24. neutrophils
25. impaired fertility

Exercise 6: Labeling

A.

Overview of Acute Radiation Lethality

Stage	Dose Gy (rad)	Average Survival Time	Signs and Symptoms
1. Prodromal	1 (100)	—	Nausea, vomiting, diarrhea, fatigue, leukopenia
2. Latent	1-100 (100-10,000)	—	None
3. Hematopoietic	1-10 (100-1000)	6-8 wk (doses over 2 Gy)	Nausea; vomiting; diarrhea; decrease in number of red blood cells, white blood cells, and platelets in the circulating blood; hemorrhage; infection
4. Gastrointestinal	6-10 (600-1000)	3-10 days	Severe nausea, vomiting, diarrhea, fever, fatigue, loss of appetite, lethargy, anemia, leukopenia, hemorrhage, infection, electrolytic imbalance, and emaciation
5. Cerebrovascular	50 and above (5000 and above)	Several hours to 2 or 3 days	Same as hematopoietic and gastrointestinal, excessive nervousness, confusion, lack of coordination, loss of vision, a burning sensation of the skin, loss of consciousness, disorientation, shock, periods of agitation alternating with stupor, edema, loss of equilibrium, meningitis, prostration, respiratory distress, vasculitis, coma

B.

Male:

1. Spermatogonia 2. Spermatocyte 3. Spermatid 4. Sperm

Female:

1. Primordial follicle 2. Mature follicle 3. Corpus luteum 4. Ovum

C.

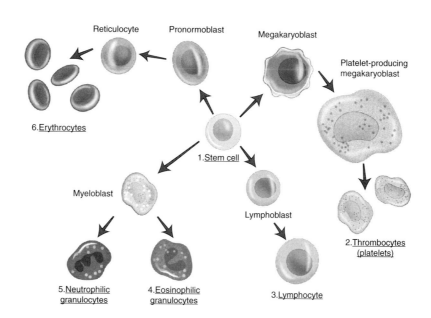

Exercise 7: Short Answer

1. Numerous laboratory animal studies and data from observation of some irradiated human populations provide substantial evidence of the consequences of high dose radiation exposure.
2. During the explosion, several tons of burning graphite, uranium dioxide fuel, and other contaminants such as cesium-137, iodine-131, and plutonium-239 were ejected vertically into the atmosphere in a 3-mile-high radioactive plume of intense heat.
3. ARS manifests in four major response stages: prodromal or initial stage, latent period, manifest illness, and recovery or death.
4. The three forms of ARS are hematopoietic syndrome (bone marrow syndrome), gastrointestinal syndrome, and cerebrovascular syndrome.
5. When the cells of the lymphatic system are damaged, the body loses some of its ability to combat infection. Because the number of platelets also decreases with loss of bone marrow function, the body loses a corresponding amount of its blood-clotting ability. This makes the body more susceptible to hemorrhage.
6. A bone marrow transplant is not an absolute cure for patients with hematopoietic syndrome because many individuals undergoing bone marrow transplant die of burns or other radiation-induced damage they sustained before the transplanted stem cells have had a chance to support recovery.
7. Some of the symptoms of the cerebrovascular syndrome are excessive nervousness, confusion, severe nausea, vomiting, diarrhea, loss of vision, a burning sensation of the skin, and loss of consciousness.
8. The techniques used to study and observe the chromosomes of each human cell have greatly contributed to genetic analysis and radiation genetics, leading to numerous observations on radiation-induced chromosome damage.
9. If there is a decrease in the number of highly radiosensitive stem cells in bone marrow as a consequence of irradiation, this decrease will manifest itself as a decrease in the number of mature circulating blood cells, thus indicating radiation damage in the bone marrow.
10. If both oxygenated and hypoxic cells receive a comparable dose of low-LET radiation, the oxygenated cells are more severely damaged, but those that survive repair themselves and recover from the injury. Even though they are less severely damaged, the hypoxic cells do not repair and recover as efficiently.
11. The radiation dose required to cause a particular syndrome and the average survival time are the most important measures used to quantify human radiation lethality.
12. When the cells of the lymphatic system are damaged by ionizing radiation, the body loses some of its ability to combat infection.
13. When shedding of the outer layer of skin occurs after reception of higher radiation doses, it generally manifests itself first as moist desquamation, and then dry desquamation may develop.
14. The goal of orthovoltage radiation therapy treatment was to deposit the radiant energy at a predetermined specific location within the tumor while sparing as much as possible the healthy surrounding tissue.
15. Most lethal dose (LD) data represent an estimate of the role played by radiation in fatalities that involved other factors. Specifications of lethal effects are further complicated by the medical treatment that the patient may receive during the prodromal and latent stages, before many of the symptoms of ARS appear. When medical treatment is given promptly, the patient is supported through initial symptoms, but the question of long-term survival may be delayed. Thus survival over a 60-day period may be a more relevant indicator of outcome for humans than survival over a 30-day period. This is the reason LD 50/60 for humans may be more accurate.

Exercise 8: General Discussion or Opinion Questions

The questions in this exercise are intended to allow students to express their knowledge and understanding of the subject matter covered in this chapter. Because the answers may vary, determination of an answer's acceptability is left to the discretion of the instructor.

Post-Test

1. early effects
2. Hematopoietic syndrome, gastrointestinal syndrome, cerebrovascular syndrome
3. prodromal, latent period, manifest illness, recovery or death
4. B
5. LD 50/30
6. cumulative
7. D
8. C
9. C
10. Nonstochastic (deterministic) somatic effects are biologic somatic effects of ionizing radiation that can be directly related to the dose received. These cell-killing effects exhibit a threshold dose below which the effect does not normally occur and above which the severity of the biologic damage increases as the dose increases.
11. Metaphase
12. Without effective physical monitoring devices, biologic criteria such as the occurrence of nausea and vomiting played an important role in the identification of radiation casualties in the first 2 days after the accident at the Chernobyl nuclear power plant.
13. gastrointestinal
14. 3 to 4 Gy (300 to 400 rad)
15. Karyotype
16. 0.1, 10, 2, 200, 5, 6, 500, 600
17. 0.1, 10
18. Cells of the hematopoietic system all develop from a single precursor cell, the pluripotential stem cell.
19. 50, 500
20. bone marrow syndrome

Chapter 8

Exercise 1: Crossword Puzzle

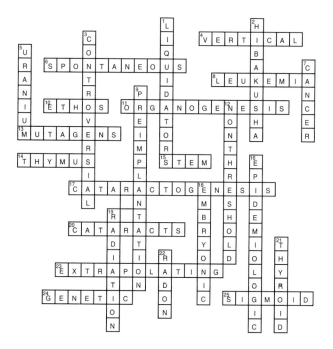

Exercise 2: Matching

1. L	6. N	11. U	16. F	21. B
2. E	7. D	12. H	17. Q	22. W
3. S	8. G	13. O	18. X	23. C
4. K	9. J	14. Y	19. P	24. R
5. A	10. I	15. V	20. T	25. M

Exercise 3: Multiple Choice

1. A	6. D	11. A	16. D	21. D
2. B	7. D	12. C	17. A	22. D
3. B	8. D	13. A	18. D	23. A
4. C	9. D	14. C	19. B	24. B
5. B	10. C	15. C	20. A	25. A

Exercise 4: True or False

1. T
2. F (nonthreshold relationship)
3. F (nonthreshold)
4. T
5. T
6. F (It is difficult to distinguish radiation-induced cancer by its physical appearance because it does not appear different from cancers caused by other agents.)
7. T
8. F (approximately 10%)
9. T
10. F (carcinogenesis)
11. F (Many cases of radiation-induced skin cancer among early radiation workers in the early 1900s have been documented.)
12. T
13. F (Technologists who entered the medical radiation industry before 1950 have demonstrated a somewhat higher risk of dying from leukemia compared with individuals who entered the workforce in 1950 or later.)
14. F (No conclusive proof exists.)
15. T
16. T
17. T
18. T
19. F (Survivors have demonstrated late deterministic and stochastic effects of ionizing radiation.)
20. T
21. T
22. F (Currently, evidence of radiation-induced genetic effects has not been observed in persons employed in diagnostic imaging or in patients undergoing radiologic examinations.)
23. F (Cancer is the most important late somatic effect caused by exposure to ionizing radiation.)
24. T
25. T

Exercise 5: Fill in the Blank

1. somatic, genetic
2. linear, threshold
3. overestimate, underestimate
4. natural, irradiated
5. risk, low
6. months, years
7. cancers
8. calcium
9. cellular
10. breast
11. 1.56, 156
12. Thorotrast, reticuloendothelial
13. malignancy
14. thyroid
15. 4:1, 10:1
16. leukemia
17. cancer-causing
18. follow-up studies
19. thyroid, iodine
20. reconstructing
21. leukemia
22. lens
23. radiosensitive, damaged
24. first, stem
25. death

Exercise 6: Labeling

A.

B.

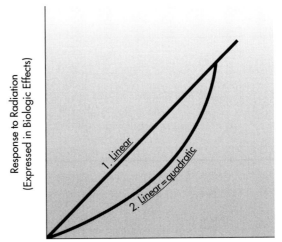

C. Late Somatic Effects

Late Nonstochastic Somatic Effects
1. Cataract formation
2. Fibrosis
3. Organ atrophy
4. Loss of parenchymal cells
5. Reduced fertility
6. Sterility

Late Stochastic Somatic Effects
7. Cancer
8. Embryologic effects (birth effects)

Exercise 7: Short Answers

1. With reference to ionizing radiation, if a threshold exists between the radiation dose and a biologic response, this means that below a certain radiation level or dose, no biologic effects are observed. Biologic effects are observed only when the threshold level or dose is reached. A nonthreshold relationship means that any radiation dose will produce a biologic effect. No radiation dose is believed to be absolutely safe.

2. Laboratory experiments on animals and data from human populations observed after acute high doses of radiation provided the foundation for a linear threshold curve of radiation dose-response.

3. Epidemiologic studies consist of observation and statistical analysis of data, such as the incidence of disease within groups of people. Such studies include the risk of radiation-induced cancer. The incident rates at which these malignancies occur as a consequence of irradiation are determined by comparing the natural incidence of cancer occurring in a human population with the incidence of cancer occurring in an irradiated population. Risk factors are then determined for the general human population.

4. To minimize the possibility of genetic effects in those persons engaged in the practice of medical imaging and in patients, gonadal shielding must be effectively used and all radiation exposure must be maintained ALARA (as low as reasonably achievable).

5. Using all data available on high radiation exposure, members of the scientific and medical communities have determined that three categories of health effects require study at low-level exposures: cancer induction, damage to the unborn from irradiation in utero, and genetic effects.

6. Three major types of late somatic effects are carcinogenesis, cataractogenesis, and embryologic effects (birth defects).
7. Evidence of human radiation cataractogenesis comes from observation of small groups of people who accidentally received substantial doses to the eyes. These groups include Japanese atomic bomb survivors, nuclear physicists working with cyclotrons from 1932 to 1960, and patients undergoing radiotherapy who received significantly high exposures to the eyes during treatment.
8. Fetal radiosensitivity decreases as gestation progresses. Hence, during the second and third trimesters, the developing fetus is less sensitive to ionizing radiation exposure. However, even in these later trimesters, congenital abnormalities and functional disorders such as sterility may be caused by radiation exposure. Leukemia also may be induced by exposure to radiation during the second and third trimesters.
9. Mutagens, such as ionizing radiation, can increase the incidence of mutations that occur as part of the natural order of events.
10. Researchers commonly use two models for extrapolation of risk from high-dose to low-dose data. These are the linear and linear-quadratic models.
11. The only evidence that ionizing radiation causes genetic effects comes from extensive experiments with fruit flies and mice at high radiation doses.
12. Point mutations (genetic mutations at the molecular level) may be either dominant (probably expressed in the offspring) or recessive (probably not expressed for several generations). Radiation is thought to cause primarily recessive mutations, if any.
13. Animal studies of radiation-induced genetic effects have led to the development of the doubling dose concept. This dose measures the effectiveness of ionizing radiation in causing mutations.
14. Gestation in humans is divided into three stages: preimplantation, which corresponds to 0 to 9 days after conception; organogenesis, which corresponds to 10 days to 6 weeks after conception; and the fetal stage, which corresponds to 6 weeks to term.
15. Because the miners had no knowledge of the adverse effects of ionizing radiation, they did not promptly change their work clothing on returning home. Because the clothing was contaminated by radioactive material, the miners' immediate families were extremely vulnerable to radiation-induced cancers.

Exercise 8: General Discussion or Opinion Questions

The questions in this exercise are intended to allow students to express their knowledge and understanding of the subject matter covered in this chapter. Because the answers may vary, determination of an answer's acceptability is left to the discretion of the instructor.

Post-Test

1. Organogenesis
2. Cancer
3. During the embryonic stage of development
4. 8
5. Absolute risk model
6. Late nonstochastic (deterministic) somatic effects are late effects that can be directly related to the dose received and occur months or years after a high-level radiation exposure.
7. Linear nonthreshold curve
8. C
9. D
10. Risk estimates to predict cancer incidence in a population may be given in terms of absolute risk or relative risk caused by a specific exposure to ionizing radiation (over and above background exposure). Both models predict the number of excess cancers, or cancers that would not have occurred in the population in question without the exposure to ionizing radiation.
11. The sigmoid, or S-shaped S (nonlinear) threshold curve of the radiation dose-response relationship is generally used in radiation therapy to demonstrate high-dose cellular response.
12. Mutant genes cannot properly govern the cell's normal chemical reactions or properly control the sequence of amino acids in the formation of specific proteins. These incapacities result in various genetic diseases.
13. Thyroid cancer
14. The term *linear-quadratic* means that the equation that best fits the data has terms that depend on dose (linear) and also dose squared (quadratic).
15. Ionizing radiation can induce genetic damage by altering the essential base coding sequence of DNA.
16. Spontaneous mutations
17. greatest
18. With reference to ionizing radiation, the term *threshold* means that no biologic effects are observed below a certain radiation level, or dose. Biologic effects are observed only when the threshold level, or dose, is reached.
19. 2, 200
20. Thyroid cancer is considered the most pronounced health consequence of the radiation accident at the Chernobyl nuclear power plant.

Chapter 9

Exercise 1: Crossword Puzzle

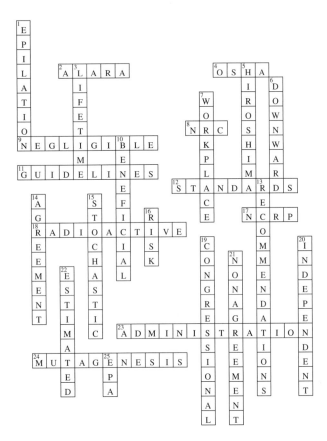

Exercise 2: Matching

1. X
2. N
3. T
4. G
5. R
6. J
7. Q
8. P
9. B
10. I
11. C
12. S
13. M
14. D
15. K
16. U
17. O
18. V
19. E
20. H
21. Y
22. F
23. A
24. L
25. W

Exercise 3: Multiple Choice

1. B
2. D
3. B
4. D
5. A
6. D
7. A
8. A
9. D
10. A
11. C
12. B
13. A
14. C
15. B
16. A
17. C
18. B
19. D
20. D
21. A
22. D
23. D
24. B
25. B

Exercise 4: True or False

1. F (It does not.)
2. T
3. T
4. F (It does not.)
5. T
6. F (do need to have an effective radiation safety program)
7. T
8. T
9. F (It is not; it conducts an ongoing electronic product radiation control program.)
10. T
11. T
12. T
13. F (It does not, the Environmental Protection Agency [EPA] does.)
14. T
15. T
16. T
17. F (The embryo-fetus is particularly sensitive.)
18. F (Effective dose limits do not include background radiation or exposure acquired when a worker undergoing medical imaging procedures.)
19. T
20. F (an active participant)
21. T
22. F (The Right-to-Know Act requires employers to evaluate their workplace for hazardous agents and provide training and written information to their employees.)
23. T
24. T
25. T

Exercise 5: Fill in the Blank

1. previous, existing, new
2. dose limits
3. nongovernmental, nonprofit
4. biologic, risk
5. radon
6. radioactive
7. radiation safety
8. dose limits
9. optimization
10. stochastic
11. 1, 0.1
12. risk
13. random
14. mutations
15. linear, linear-quadratic
16. risk
17. greater
18. 0.4, 40
19. 8, 15
20. cancer, genetic
21. whole body
22. nonoccupationally
23. same
24. external, internal
25. 50, 5, 10

Exercise 6: Labeling

A.

Summary of Radiation Protection Standards Organizations

Organization	Function
1. ICRP	Evaluates information on biologic effects of radiation and provides radiation protection guidance through general recommendations on occupational and public dose limits
2. NCRP	Reviews regulations formulated by the ICRP and decides ways to include those recommendations in U.S. radiation protection criteria
3. UNSCEAR	Evaluates human and environmental ionizing radiation exposure and derives radiation risk assessments from epidemiologic data and research conclusions; provides information to organizations such as the ICRP for evaluation
4. NAS/NRC-BEIR	Reviews studies of biologic effects of ionizing radiation and risk assessment and provides the information to organizations such as the ICRP for evaluation

B.

Summary of U.S. Regulatory Agencies

Agency	Function
1. NRC	Oversees the nuclear energy industry; enforces radiation protection standards; publishes its rules and regulations in Title 10 of the U.S. Code of Federal Regulations; enters into written agreements with state governments, permitting the state to license and regulate the use of radioisotopes and certain other material within that state
2. Agreement states	Enforces radiation protection regulations through their respective health departments
3. EPA	Facilitates the development and enforcement of regulations pertaining to the control of radiation in the environment
4. FDA	Conducts an ongoing product radiation control program, regulating the design and manufacture of electronic products, including x-ray equipment
5. OSHA	Functions as a monitoring agency in places of employment, predominantly in industry

Summary of the National Council on Radiation Protection and Measurements (NCRP) Recommendations*†
(NCRP Report No. 116)

A. Occupational exposures‡		
1. Effective dose limits		
a. Annual	1. <u>50</u> mSv	(<u>5</u> rem)
b. Cumulative	2. <u>10</u> mSv × age	<u>1</u> rem × age
2. Equivalent dose annual limits for tissues and organs		
a. Lens of eye	3. <u>150</u> mSv	(<u>15</u> rem)
b. Localized areas of the skin, hands, and feet	4. <u>500</u> mSv	(<u>50</u> rem)
B. Guidance for emergency occupational exposure‡ (see Section 14, NCRP Report No. 116)		
C. Public exposures (annual)		
1. Effective dose limit, continuous or frequent exposure‡	5. <u>1</u> mSv	(<u>0.1</u> rem)
2. Effective dose limit, infrequent exposure‡	6. <u>5</u> mSv	(<u>0.5</u> rem)
3. Equivalent dose limits for tissues and organs‡		
a. Lens of eye	7. <u>15</u> mSv	(<u>1.5</u> rem)
b. Localized areas of the skin, hands, and feet	8. <u>50</u> mSv	(<u>5</u> rem)
4. Remedial action for natural sources		
a. Effective dose (excluding radon)	9. >$\underline{5}$ mSv	(>$\underline{0.5}$ rem)
b. Exposure to radon and its decay products§	10. >26 J/(s m^{-3})ǁ	(<u>13</u> WLM)
D. Education and training exposures (annual)‡		
1. Effective dose limit	11. <u>1</u> mSv	(<u>0.1</u> rem)
2. Equivalent dose limit for tissues and organs		
a. Lens of eye	12. <u>15</u> mSv	(<u>1.5</u> rem)
b. Localized areas of the skin, hands, and feet	13. <u>50</u> mSv	(<u>5</u> rem)
E. Embryo-fetus exposures‡		
1. Equivalent dose limit		
a. Monthly	14. <u>0.5</u> mSv	(<u>0.05</u> rem)
b. Entire gestation	15. <u>5.0</u> mSv	(<u>0.5</u> rem)
F. Negligible individual dose (annual)‡	16. <u>0.01</u> mSv	(<u>0.001</u> rem)

*Excluding medical exposures.
†See Tables 4.2 and 5.1 in NCRP Report No. 116 for recommendations on radiation weighting factors and tissue weighting factors, respectively.
‡Sum of external and internal exposures, excluding doses from natural sources.
§WLM stands for working level month and refers to a cumulative exposure for a working month (170 h). As applied to radon and its daughter products, 1 WLM represents the cumulative exposure experienced in a 170-h period resulting from a radon concentration of 100 pCi/L. The occupational limit for miners is 4 WLM per year, which results in a dose equivalent of approximately 0.15 Sv (15 rem) per year.
ǁA measure of the rate of release of energy (joules per second) by radon and its decay products per unit volume of air (cubic meters).

Exercise 7: Short Answer

1. Exposure of the general public, patients, and radiation workers to ionizing radiation must be limited to minimize the risk of harmful biologic effects.
2. Medical imaging professionals must be familiar with previous, existing, and new guidelines because they share the responsibility for patient safety from radiation exposure and also are subject to such exposure in the performance of their duties. By keeping themselves informed, they will be more conscious of good radiation safety practices.
3. Four major organizations that are responsible for evaluating the relationship between radiation equivalent dose (EqD) and induced biologic effects are the International Commission on Radiological Protection (ICRP); the National Council on Radiation Protection and Measurements (NCRP); the United Nations Scientific Committee on the Effects of Atomic Radiation (UNSCEAR); and the National Academy of Sciences/National Research Council Committee on the Biological Effects of Ionizing Radiation (NAS/NRC-BEIR).
4. Five U.S. regulatory agencies are responsible for enforcing radiation protection standards to safeguard the general public, patients, and occupationally exposed personnel: the Nuclear Regulatory Commission (NRC); states that have signed an NRC agreement; the Environmental Protection Agency (EPA); the Food and Drug Administration (FDA); and the Occupational Safety and Health Administration (OSHA).
5. The NRC mandates that a radiation safety committee (RSC) be established for the health care facility to assist in the development of radiation safety programs. This committee provides guidance for the program and facilitates its ongoing operation.
6. The necessary training and experience for a radiation safety officer (RSO) are described in § 10 CFR 35.50 and § 10 CFR 35.900 of the Code of Federal Regulations. Three training pathways are specified: (1) certification by one of the professional boards approved by the NRC, (2) didactic and work experience as described in detail in the regulations, and (3) identification as an authorized user, authorized medical physicist, or authorized nuclear physicist on the license, with experience in the types of use for which the individual has RSO responsibility.
7. To define the designation *as low as reasonably achievable (ALARA)*, health care facilities usually adopt investigation levels, defined as Level I and Level II. In the United States these levels traditionally are one tenth to three tenths the applicable regulatory limits.
8. Radiation protection has two explicit objectives: (1) to prevent any clinically important radiation-induced nonstochastic (deterministic) effect from occurring by adhering to dose limits that are beneath the threshold levels and (2) to limit the risk of stochastic responses to a conservative level as weighted against societal needs, values, benefits acquired, and economic considerations.

9. Occupational risk associated with radiation exposure may be equated with occupational risk in other industries that are generally considered reasonably safe (i.e., about 10^{-4} to 10^{-6} annually, meaning an excess cancer risk of one chance in 10,000 to one chance in 1 million per year). The risk generally is estimated to be a 2.5% chance of a fatal accident over an entire career.
10. The Consumer-Patient Radiation Health and Safety Act of 1981 carries no legal penalty for noncompliance; therefore several states simply have not responded with appropriate legislation.
11. When ionizing radiation damages reproductive cells, mutations may develop that could have deleterious consequences in subsequent generations. An example of this is effects on offspring caused by irradiation of reproductive cells (sperm and ova) before conception. This effect is called *mutagenesis*.
12. Two all-inclusive categories that encompass the radiation-induced responses of serious concern in radiation protection programs are nonstochastic (deterministic) effects and stochastic (probabilistic) effects.
13. The purpose of the Consumer-Patient Radiation Health and Safety Act of 1981 is to ensure that standard medical and dental radiologic procedures adhere to rigorous safety precautions and standards.
14. The EPA was established on December 2, 1970, to bring several agencies into one organization that would be responsible for protecting the health of human beings and for safeguarding the natural environment.
15. Exposure linearity is defined as consistency in output radiation intensity at a selected KVp setting while changing from one milliamperage and time combination to another.

Exercise 8: General Discussion or Opinion Questions

The questions in this exercise are intended to allow students to express their knowledge and understanding of the subject matter covered in this chapter. Because the answers may vary, determination of an answer's acceptability is left to the discretion of the instructor.

Exercise 9: Calculation Problems

1. EqD = 10 mSv × Age (yr)
   EqD = 10 mSv × 54
   EqD = 540 mSv
2. EqD = Age in rem
   EqD = 54 rem
3. EqD = 10 mSv × Age (yr)
   EqD = 10 mSv × 46
   EqD = 460 mSv
4. EqD = Age in rem
   EqD = 46 rem
5. EqD = 10 mSv × Age (yr)
   EqD = 10 mSv × 33
   EqD = 330 mSv
6. EqD = Age in rem
   EqD = 33 rem
7. EqD = 10 mSv × Age (yr)
   EqD = 10 mSv × 25
   EqD = 250 mSv
8. EqD = Age in rem
   EqD = 25 rem
9. EqD = 10 mSv × Age (yr)
   EqD = 10 mSv × 18
   EqD = 180 mSv
10. EqD = Age in rem
    EqD = 18 rem

Post-Test

1. In the medical industry, with reference to the radiation sciences, risk is the possibility of inducing a radiogenic cancer or genetic defect after irradiation.
2. national security
3. Occupational Safety and Health Administration (OSHA)
4. The radiation safety officer (RSO)
5. EqD = 10 mSv × Age (yr)
   EqD = 10 mSv × 39
   EqD = 390 mSv
6. EqD = Age in rem
   EqD = 39 rem
7. Effective dose-limiting system
8. ALARA is the acronym for *as low as reasonably achievable*.
9. B
10. C
11. estimated
12. linear nonthreshold
13. Occupational risk in other industries generally considered reasonably safe
14. The essential concept underlying radiation protection is that any organ in the human body is vulnerable to damage from exposure to ionizing radiation.
15. The NCRP now recommends an equivalent dose limit of 5 mSv (0.5 rem) during the entire period of gestation.
16. 50 mSv (5 rem)
17. Accounting for tissue weighting factors is important because various tissues and organs do not have the same degree of sensitivity.
18. effective
19. Radiation hormesis is the hypothesis that a positive effect exists for certain populations that are continuously exposed to moderate levels of radiation.
20. Internal action limits are established by health care facilities to trigger an investigation to uncover the reasons for any unusual high exposures received by individual staff members.

Chapter 10

Exercise 1: Crossword Puzzle

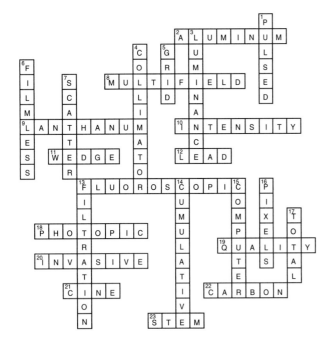

Exercise 2: Matching

1. N	6. O	11. U	16. A	21. V
2. I	7. Y	12. C	17. T	22. D
3. L	8. F	13. S	18. G	23. X
4. J	9. P	14. H	19. Q	24. B
5. K	10. E	15. W	20. M	25. R

Exercise 3: Multiple Choice

1. D	6. A	11. B	16. D	21. A
2. B	7. A	12. C	17. A	22. B
3. A	8. D	13. C	18. B	23. B
4. A	9. D	14. A	19. C	24. A
5. C	10. A	15. B	20. C	25. D

Exercise 4: True or False

1. T
2. F (The radiographer must ensure that collimation is adequate by collimating the radiographic beam so that it is no larger than the image receptor.)
3. F (These are x-ray beam limitation devices.)
4. T
5. F (inherent amounts to 0.5 mm aluminum equivalent)
6. T
7. F (It is important in mammography.)
8. F (Rare earth elements used in intensifying screens have high atomic numbers ranging from 57 to 71.)
9. T
10. T
11. F (Europium-activated barium fluorohalide is the most commonly used photostimulable phosphor in computed radiography imaging plates.)
12. T
13. F (Radiation shielding requirements are decreased because of the reduction of x-radiation in the environment.)
14. F (The patient dose increases.)
15. F (It is not acceptable.)
16. F (In CR imaging the practice of overexposing patients to possibly avoid repeat radiographic exposures is unethical and unacceptable.)
17. T
18. T
19. T
20. F (the use of carbon fiber)
21. T
22. F (When compared with conventional screen-film systems, the photostimulable phosphor in the CR imaging plate is much more sensitive to scatter radiation before and after it is sensitized through exposure to a radiographic beam. Because of this increased sensitivity, a radiographic grid may be used more frequently during CR imaging.)
23. F (2 mm lead equivalent)
24. T
25. T

Exercise 5: Fill in the Blank

1. manufacturer, federal
2. limitation
3. under
4. dead-man, incapacitated
5. decreases
6. latitude, less
7. center
8. technique
9. wedge
10. electronic
11. same
12. distance
13. image matrix
14. mAs
15. quality
16. quantum mottle
17. reduces
18. increase
19. density
20. workstations
21. mispositioning
22. dose reduction
23. multifield
24. entrance, exit
25. energized

Exercise 6: Labeling

A.

B.

From Bushong SC: *Radiologic science for technologists: physics, biology and protection*, ed 9, St. Louis, 2008, Elsevier.

C.

HVL Required by the Radiation Control for Health and Safety Act of 1968 and Detailed by the Bureau of Radiological Health* in 1980

Peak Kilovoltage	Minimum Required HVL in Millimeters of Aluminum
30	1. 0.3
40	2. 0.4
50	3. 1.2
60	4. 1.3
70	5. 1.5
80	6. 2.3
90	7. 2.5
100	8. 2.7
110	9. 3.0
120	10. 3.2

*The Bureau of Radiological Health changed its name to the Center for Devices and Radiological Health in 1982.

Exercise 7: Short Answer

1. If adequate filtration were not present, very-low–energy photons (20 keV or lower) would enter the patient and be almost totally absorbed in the body, increasing the patient's radiation dose but contributing nothing to the image process.
2. The first set of shutters in the collimator, the upper shutters, are mounted as close as possible to the x-ray tube window to reduce the amount of off-focus, or stem, radiation coming from the primary beam and exiting at various angles from the x-ray tube window. This radiation can never be completely eliminated because the metal shutters cannot be placed immediately beneath the actual focal spot of the x-ray tube, but placing the upper shutters as close as possible to the tube window can reduce it significantly. This practice reduces patient exposure resulting from off-focus radiation.
3. In general diagnostic radiology, aluminum (atomic number 13) is the medal most widely selected as a filter material because it effectively removes low-energy (soft) x-rays from a polyenergetic (heterogeneous) x-ray beam without severely decreasing the x-ray beam intensity. Also, aluminum is lightweight, sturdy, relatively inexpensive, and readily available.
4. Because HVL is a measure of beam quality or effective energy of the x-ray beam, a certain minimal HVL is required at a given peak kilovoltage.
5. Either each image should be monitored by an independent quality control technologist at a separate monitor, or a quality control system should exist whereby the number of images per examination is compared with the number ordered for each technologist.
6. With cone vision the radiologist does not need to adapt his or her eyes to darkness to perform the examination, thereby saving time. Cone vision also significantly improves visual acuity, thereby permitting the radiologist to better discriminate between small structures.
7. Inherent filtration includes the glass envelope encasing the x-ray tube, the insulating oil surrounding the tube, and the glass window in the x-ray tube housing.
8. Three reasons for high radiation exposure during interventional procedures performed by a physician who is not a radiologist include the following: (1) the fluoroscopic tube may be operated for longer periods in continuous rather than pulsed mode; (2) the protective curtain, or floating shields, on the stationary fluoroscopic equipment's image intensifier may not be used as a means of protection; and (3) cine is extensively used as a recording medium.
9. The FDA has recommended that a notation be placed in the patient's record if skin dose in the range of 1 to 2 Gy (100 to 200 rad) is received.
10. The use of a pulsed progressive system for digital fluoroscopy results in decreased patient dose.
11. Because filtration absorbs some of the photons in the radiographic beam, it decreases the overall intensity (amount, or quantity) of radiation. The remaining photons, however, are as a whole more penetrating and therefore less likely to be absorbed in body tissue.
12. Added filtration is located outside the glass window of the x-ray tube housing, above the collimator shutters.
13. The housing enclosing the x-ray tube must be so constructed so that the leakage radiation measured at a distance of 1 m (3.3 feet) from the x-ray source does not exceed 100 mR/h (2.58×10^{-5} C/kg)/h when the tube is operated at its highest voltage at the highest current that allows continuous operation.
14. The control panel must be located behind a suitable protective barrier that has a radiation-absorbent window that permits observation of the patient during any procedure.
15. The thickness of a radiographic examination tabletop must be uniform, and the tabletop must also be as radiolucent as possible, so that it will absorb only a minimal amount of radiation, thereby reducing the patient's radiation dose.
16. It is also known as a *trough filter*.
17. Eleven procedures involving extended fluoroscopic time are (1) percutaneous transluminal angioplasty, (2) radiofrequency cardiac catheter ablation, (3) vascular embolization, (4) stent and filter placement, (5) thrombolytic and fibrinolytic procedures, (6) percutaneous transhepatic cholangiography, (7) endoscopic retrograde cholangiopancreatography, (8) transjugular intrahepatic portosystemic shunt, (9) percutaneous nephrostomy, (10) biliary drainage, and (11) urinary or biliary stone removal.
18. The resettable cumulative timing device on fluoroscopic equipment times the x-ray beam-on time and sounds an audible alarm or temporarily interrupts the exposure after the fluoroscope has been activated for 5 min. It makes the radiologist aware of the length of time for which the patient receives exposure for each fluoroscopic examination.
19. For dose reduction purposes, whenever possible it is best to position the C-arm so that the x-ray tube is under the patient. Scatter radiation is less intense with the x-ray tube in this position. When the tube is positioned over the patient, scatter radiation becomes more intense, and the patient dose increases accordingly.
20. Current federal standards limit entrance skin exposure rates of general-purpose intensified fluoroscopic units to a maximum of 10 roentgens (R) per minute ($10 \times 2.58 \times 10^{-4}$ coulomb [C] per kg/min).

Exercise 8: General Discussion or Opinion Questions

The questions in this exercise are intended to allow students to express their knowledge and understanding of the subject matter covered in this chapter. Because the answers may vary, determination of an answer's acceptability is left to the discretion of the instructor.

Post-Test
1. 10
2. Carbon fiber
3. protective, control
4. Light-localizing variable-aperture rectangular collimator
5. Scattered radiation is all the radiation that arises from the interaction of an x-ray beam with the atoms of a patient or any other object in the path of the beam.
6. Use of a radiographic grid results in an increase in the patient dose.
7. digital, image matrix
8. D
9. B
10. integral dose
11. quantum mottle
12. Interventional
13. mAs
14. The radiologist should use the practice of intermittent, or pulsed, fluoroscopy to reduce the overall length of exposure.
15. D
16. Patient-image intensifier distance should be as short as possible.
17. pixels
18. Radiographic equipment must have a source-to–image receptor distance (SID) indicator.
19. D
20. unethical, unacceptable

Chapter 11

Exercise 1: Crossword Puzzle

Exercise 2: Matching
1. N
2. J
3. L
4. Y
5. M
6. O
7. W
8. K
9. P
10. E
11. X
12. D
13. S
14. H
15. G
16. A
17. U
18. C
19. Q
20. F
21. V
22. R
23. I
24. B
25. T

Exercise 3: Multiple Choice
1. D
2. B
3. B
4. A
5. C
6. A
7. D
8. D
9. D
10. A
11. D
12. D
13. D
14. A
15. C
16. B
17. D
18. A
19. C
20. D
21. B
22. A
23. C
24. C
25. D

Exercise 4: True or False
1. T
2. F (Patients do need to be given the opportunity.)
3. F (They will deteriorate over time.)
4. T
5. F (An air gap technique removes scatter radiation by using an increased object-to–image receptor distance)
6. T
7. F (They need to be selectively shielded.)
8. F (may be reduced as much as 90% to 95%)
9. T
10. T
11. F (higher kVp, lower mAs)
12. T
13. F (A gonadal shield should be a secondary protective measure, not a substitute for an adequate collimated beam.)
14. F (Dose reduction in mammography can be achieved by limiting the number of projections taken.)
15. F (It is not acceptable.)
16. F (The radiation dose to the breast of a young patient may be further reduced by performing the scoliosis examination with the x-ray beam entering the posterior surface of the patient's body instead of the anterior surface.)
17. T
18. T
19. T
20. F (Axillary projections should be done only on request of the radiologist.)
21. T
22. F (It is 100 times the exit dose.)
23. F (Patient dose increases.)
24. T
25. T

Exercise 5: Fill in the Blank

1. reduction, protective, minimize
2. Holistic, effective
3. cooperate
4. poor
5. reproductive
6. female, male
7. reduces
8. symphysis pubis
9. remote, over
10. beam-defining
11. milliampere-second
12. Computed tomography
13. increases, decreases
14. clinical interest
15. 0.20, 20
16. 90, 95
17. shadow
18. minimal
19. 50
20. additional
21. less
22. mean marrow
23. placement, radiosensitive
24. helical
25. pregnancy, menstrual period

Exercise 6: Labeling

A.

Technical Exposure Factor Considerations

1. Mass per unit volume of tissue of the area of clinical interest
2. Effective atomic numbers and electron densities of the tissues involved
3. Film-screen combination or other type of image receptor
4. Source-to–image receptor distance (SID)
5. Type and quantity of filtration employed
6. Type of x-ray generator used (single- phase, three-phase, or high-frequency)
7. Balance of radiographic density and contrast required

B.

C.

Benefits of a Repeat Analysis Program

1. The program increases awareness among staff and student radiographers of the need to produce optimal-quality recorded images.
2. Radiographers generally become more careful in producing their radiographic images because they are aware that the images are being reviewed.
3. When the repeat analysis program identifies problems or concerns, in-service education programs covering these specific topics may be designed for imaging personnel.

Exercise 7: Short Answer

1. During a diagnostic x-ray procedure, radiographers can limit the patient's exposure to ionizing radiation by employing appropriate radiation reduction techniques and by using protective devices that minimize radiation exposure. Patient exposure can be substantially reduced by using proper body or part immobilization, motion reduction techniques, appropriate beam limitation devices and adequate filtration of the x-ray beam, and gonadal or other specific area shielding. Selection of suitable technical exposure factors, used in conjunction with either high-speed film-screen combinations or computer-generated digital images, correct radiographic film processing techniques or appropriate digital image processing, and the elimination of repeat radiographic exposures, can also contribute significantly to limiting patient exposure.
2. The radiographer must achieve a balance in technical radiographic exposure factors to ensure the presence of adequate information in the recorded image and minimize patient dose.
3. The four basic types of gonadal shielding devices that can be used during a diagnostic x-ray procedure are flat contact shields, shadow shields, shaped contact shields, and clear lead shields.
4. Poorly processed radiographs offer inadequate diagnostic information, leading to repeat exposures and unnecessary patient radiation exposure.
5. Protective shielding is a structure or device made of certain materials (e.g., concrete, lead, or lead-impregnated material) that will adequately attenuate ionizing radiation.
6. For an air gap technique to be performed, the image receptor is placed 6 to 10 inches (15 to 25 cm) from the patient, and the x-ray tube is placed approximately 10 to 12 feet (2.7 to 3.6 m) away from the image receptor. The scattered x-rays produced in the patient (the source of the scatter) are disseminated in many directions at acute angles to the primary beam when the radiographic exposure is made. Because of this and the increased distance between the anatomy imaged and the image receptor, a higher percentage of the scattered x-rays produced are then less likely to strike the image receptor. The air gap method results in an adequate grid-type scatter cleanup effect. In general, the use of an air gap technique requires the selection of technical exposure factors that are comparable to those used with an 8:1 ratio grid. Therefore when the patient dose is compared with a nongrid technique, it is higher. When compared with the patient dose resulting from the use of a midratio grid (8:1), the dose from an air gap technique is about the same as with the midratio grid.
7. Before ordering a radiologic examination, the referring physician must determine whether the benefit to the patient in terms of medical information gained sufficiently justifies subjecting the patient to the risk of the absorbed radiation resulting from the procedure.

8. The five layers of the epidermis are: (1) the horny, or outer, layer; (2) translucent, or clear, layer; (3) granular layer; (4) prickle cell layer; and (5) germinal, or basal, cell layer.
9. Four ways to specify the amount of radiation a patient receives from a diagnostic imaging procedure are entrance skin exposure (ESE), skin dose, gonadal dose, and bone marrow dose.
10. Direct patient shielding is not typically used in computed tomography (CT). Because of the rotational nature of the exposure, a shield is no more effective than the collimators that already exist on the device. Because the beam is so tightly collimated to the slice thickness, exposure to the anatomy outside the field of view is usually caused only by internal scatter. Generally in CT, anatomy does not appear in the primary x-ray beam unless it is part of the intended field of view.
11. Members in a population who cannot bear children (e.g., those who are beyond reproductive years) have no genetic impact and would not be included in genetically significant dose considerations.
12. It is strongly recommended that the result of a pregnancy test be obtained before the pelvis is irradiated.
13. Experts advise yearly mammographic screening for women 50 years of age or older.
14. Good communication encourages reduction in anxiety and emotional stress, enhances the professional image of the radiographer as a person who cares about the patient's well-being, and increases the chance for successful completion of the x-ray examination.
15. Six x-ray procedures now considered nonessential are (1) a chest x-ray examination on scheduled admission to the hospital; (2) a chest x-ray examination as part of a preemployment physical; (3) a lumbar spine examination as part of a preemployment physical; (4) chest x-ray studies or other unjustified x-ray examinations as part of a routine health checkup; (5) a chest x-ray examination for mass screening for tuberculosis; and (6) a whole-body multislice spiral CT screening procedure.
16. Seven categories that may be established for discarded images are (1) images too dark or too light because of inappropriate selection of technical exposure factors; (2) incorrect patient positioning; (3) incorrect centering of the radiographic beam; (4) patient motion during the radiographic exposure; (5) improper collimation of the radiographic beam; (6) presence of external foreign bodies; and (7) processing artifacts.
17. The two concerns related to patient dose in CT scanning are (1) the skin dose and (2) the dose distribution during the scanning procedure.
18. The first goal of the Alliance is to raise awareness among nonradiology users of CT. If a child is placed in a CT scanner and adult protocols are used, the child will receive a higher dose than an adult would, but the image will appear to be of acceptable quality—it will not appear overexposed as a film would. Radiologists have been aware of this for some time, and many practices have altered their protocols for pediatric patients. But as of 2007, many referring physicians and nonradiology owners of CT scanners were not aware of the problem.
19. The campaign includes dissemination of information on pediatric CT dose reduction among the various medical specialties that refer or even operate their own CT scanners. It also included the establishment of the Image Gently website.
20. A small, relatively thin pack of thermoluminescent dosimeters (TLDs) is secured to the patient's skin in the middle of the clinical area of interest and exposed during a radiographic procedure. Because lithium fluoride (LiF), the sensing material in the TLD, responds in a manner similar to human tissue when exposed to ionizing radiation, an accurate determination of surface dose can be made.

Exercise 8: General Discussion or Opinion Questions

The questions in this exercise are intended to allow students to express their knowledge and understanding of the subject matter covered in this chapter. Because the answers may vary, determination of an answer's acceptability is left to the discretion of the instructor.

Post-Test

1. Image Gently campaign
2. F. B. Reynold stated the official position of the American College of Radiology at a press conference on October 20, 1976: "Abdominal radiological exams that have been requested after full consideration of the clinical status of a patient, including the possibility of pregnancy, need not be postponed or selectively scheduled."
3. double dose
4. Direct patient shielding
5. The genetically significant dose (GSD) is the equivalent dose to the reproductive organs that, if received by every human, would be expected to bring about an identical gross genetic injury to the total population as does the sum of the actual doses received by exposed individual members of the population.
6. To protect the ovaries of a female patient, the ovarian shield should be placed approximately 1 inch (2.5 cm) medial to each palpable anterior superior iliac spine.
7. effective
8. D
9. D
10. collimated
11. posterior, anterior
12. The referring physician
13. 50
14. About 0.20 mSv (20 mrem)
15. D
16. A calculated estimate of the approximate equivalent dose to the embryo-fetus as a result of the examination should be obtained.
17. three
18. The symphysis pubis can be used to guide shield placement over the testes.
19. B
20. projections

Chapter 12

Exercise 1: Crossword Puzzle

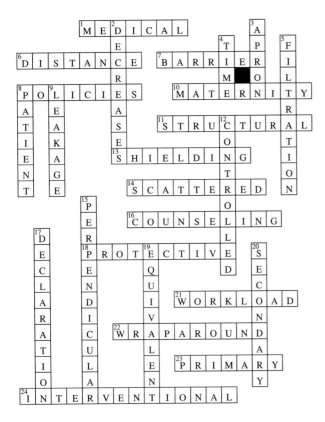

Exercise 2: Matching

1. C	6. U	11. J	16. V	21. E
2. P	7. I	12. T	17. B	22. Y
3. F	8. O	13. A	18. N	23. H
4. S	9. Q	14. G	19. X	24. D
5. K	10. L	15. R	20. M	25. W

Exercise 3: Multiple Choice

1. A	6. D	11. C	16. D	21. D
2. D	7. D	12. D	17. C	22. D
3. D	8. D	13. C	18. D	23. A
4. D	9. A	14. B	19. C	24. A
5. B	10. B	15. D	20. D	25. D

Exercise 4: True or False

1. T
2. F (Personal medical and natural background radiation exposure are not included.)
3. T
4. T
5. F (inversely proportional)
6. F (0.5 mm lead equivalency)
7. F (0.25 mm thickness of lead)
8. T
9. F (Bucky slot shielding device)
10. T
11. F (limits the methods that can be used to achieve protection)
12. T
13. F (A radiographer should never stand in the useful beam to restrain a patient during a radiographic exposure.)
14. T
15. T
16. F (primarily benefits the patient)
17. F (as a consequence of the Compton scattering process)
18. T
19. T
20. F (Diagnostic imaging department staff members who are pregnant should be able to continue performing their duties without interruption of employment if they follow radiation safety practices.)
21. F (directly proportional)
22. T
23. T
24. T
25. F (During fluoroscopic examinations, the radiographer should always wear a protective apron.)

Exercise 5: Fill in the Blank

1. equivalent dose
2. Scattered
3. decrease, reduction
4. safety
5. increased
6. Shortening
7. distance
8. shielding
9. aprons, gloves, thyroid shields
10. housing, high-tension
11. Compton scatter, Compton scatter
12. 0.5, 0.05, 5, 0.5
13. 0.5 mm, 1 mm
14. time, distance, shielding
15. four, four
16. perpendicular
17. $\frac{1}{16}$ inch, 7, 2.1
18. $\frac{1}{32}$ inch
19. 0.5 mm
20. scattered, patient, assistance
21. 0.25 mm
22. magnify
23. wraparound
24. right angles, 90, least
25. routine

Exercise 6: Labeling

A.

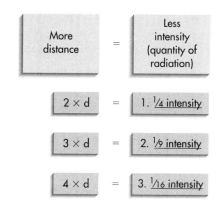

1. ¼ intensity
2. ⅑ intensity
3. ¹⁄₁₆ intensity

B.

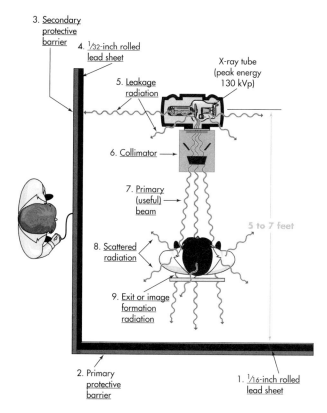

1. ¹⁄₁₆-inch rolled lead sheet
2. Primary protective barrier
3. Secondary protective barrier
4. ¹⁄₃₂-inch rolled lead sheet
5. Leakage radiation
6. Collimator
7. Primary (useful) beam
8. Scattered radiation
9. Exit or image formation radiation

C.

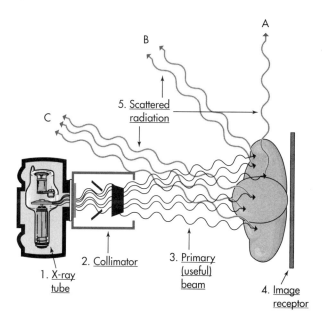

1. X-ray tube
2. Collimator
3. Primary (useful) beam
4. Image receptor
5. Scattered radiation

Exercise 7: Short Answer

1. The occupational risk for monitored diagnostic imaging personnel may be compared with the occupational risk for people employed in other industries generally considered reasonably safe, such as government and trade. These jobs have a risk of fatal accidents generally estimated to be about 1×10^{-4} yr^{-1}.
2. Lead aprons are designed to provide protection from secondary (leakage and scatter) radiation.
3. When high-speed imaging receptor systems are used, smaller radiographic exposure (less milliamperage) is required, which results in fewer x-ray photons being available to produce Compton scatter. Because of this reduction in Compton scatter, personnel exposure is decreased.
4. Most health care facilities have policies for protecting pregnant personnel from radiation. Under these policies, an imaging professional who becomes pregnant first informs her supervisor. After this voluntary "declaration" has been made, the health care facility officially recognizes the pregnancy. The facility, through its radiation safety officer, provides essential counseling and furnishes an appropriate additional monitor that should be worn at waist level during all radiation procedures.
5. The three basic principles of radiation protection are time, distance, and shielding.
6. A qualified medical physicist will determine the exact protection requirements for a particular imaging facility.
7. Protective aprons, gloves, and thyroid shields are made of lead-impregnated vinyl.
8. Diagnostic imaging personnel can substantially reduce scatter radiation to the lens of the eyes by wearing protective eyeglasses with optically clear lenses that contain a minimal lead equivalent protection of 0.35 mm. Side shields on the glasses are also available for procedures that require turning of the head. A wraparound frame containing optically clear lenses with a 0.5 mm lead equivalency is also available.
9. A lead-lined, metal, diagnostic-type protective tube housing protects both the radiographer and the patient from off-focus, or leakage, radiation by restricting the emission of x-rays to the area of the useful, or primary, beam.

10. Remote control fluoroscopic systems provide the best radiation protection for imaging personnel. These systems permit the radiologist and assisting radiographer to remain outside the fluoroscopy room at a control console located behind a protective barrier until needed. This increases imaging personnel safety because distance is used as a means of increased protection. With remote equipment, the radiologist and assisting radiographer can view the patient directly through clear protective shielding and will enter the x-ray room only when absolutely necessary to provide essential patient care or perform procedural functions.

11. Positioning of a C-arm fluoroscope with the x-ray tube over the table and the image intensifier underneath the table results in higher patient exposure and increased scatter radiation. As scatter increases, radiation exposure of all personnel in the immediate vicinity of the C-arm also increases. Therefore, just from the perspective of increased radiation safety, it is best to reverse the C-arm to place the x-ray tube under the table and the image intensifier over the table.

12. Exposure of personnel is caused by scatter radiation from the patient. During operating room procedures in which cross-table exposures are made with a mobile C-arm fluoroscope, an understanding of the patterns of x-ray scatter is particularly useful. The exposure rate caused by scatter near the entrance surface of the patient (the x-ray tube side) exceeds the exposure rate caused by scatter near the exit surface of the patient (the image intensifier side). The difference in the amount of scatter, typically a factor of 2 or 3, is caused by the higher radiation intensity at the entrance surface of the patient. Thus the location of the lower potential scatter dose is on the side of the patient away from the x-ray tube (i.e., the image intensifier side).

13. The radiologist or other interventional physician can reduce radiation exposure during a high-level-control interventional procedure by shortening the duration of the procedure, thereby decreasing fluoroscopic beam-on time; taking fewer digital and cineradiographic images; reducing the use of continuous as contrasted to pulsed mode of operation; keeping the protective curtain, if present, on the image intensifier or scatter shield in place during a procedure; and regularly using the last-image-hold feature to view the most recent fluoroscopic images. These good safety practices will substantially decrease exposure of all participating personnel and of the patient as well.

14. Because the hands and forearms of physicians performing interventional procedures can be subject to large radiation exposures if the safety protocol is not carefully followed and because sometimes this may not be possible, it is imperative that extremities be monitored. Physicians need to be aware of the recommended dose limits that have been established for the extremities. The National Council of Radiation Protection and Measurements (NCRP) currently recommends an annual equivalent dose limit to localized areas of the skin and hands of 500 mSv (50 rem). To avoid remotely approaching this limit and consequently increasing the possibility of adverse effects, protective gloves should be worn whenever possible by any physician whose hands will of necessity often be close to the fluoroscopic beam.

15. Eight radiation-absorbent barrier design considerations are (1) the mean energy of the x-ray beam that will strike the barrier; (2) whether the barrier is of a primary or secondary nature; (3) the distance from the x-ray source to a position of occupancy 1 foot (30 cm) from the barrier; (4) the workload of the unit; (5) the use factor of the unit; (6) the occupancy factor behind the barrier; (7) the intrinsic shielding (e.g., tube housing attenuation) of the x-ray unit; and (8) whether the area beyond the barrier is controlled or uncontrolled.

Exercise 8: General Discussion or Opinion Questions

The questions in this exercise are intended to allow students to express their knowledge and understanding of the subject matter covered in this chapter. Because the answers may vary, determination of an answer's acceptability is left to the discretion of the instructor.

Exercise 9: Calculation Problems

1. $\dfrac{I_1}{I_2} = \dfrac{(d_2)^2}{(d_1)^2}$

   $\dfrac{9}{I_2} = \dfrac{(6)^2}{(3)^2}$

   $\dfrac{9}{I_2} = \dfrac{36}{9}$ (cross-multiply)

   $36 I_2 = 81$
   $I_2 = 2.25\,\text{mR/h}$

2. $\dfrac{I_1}{I_2} = \dfrac{(d_2)^2}{(d_1)^2}$

   $\dfrac{5}{I_2} = \dfrac{(4)^2}{(2)^2}$

   $\dfrac{5}{I_2} = \dfrac{16}{4}$ (cross-multiply)

   $16 I_2 = 20$
   $I_2 = 1.25\,\text{mR/h}$

3. $\dfrac{I_1}{I_2} = \dfrac{(d_2)^2}{(d_1)^2}$

   $\dfrac{4}{I_2} = \dfrac{(10)^2}{(5)^2}$

   $\dfrac{4}{I_2} = \dfrac{100}{25}$ (cross-multiply)

   $100 I_2 = 100$
   $I_2 = 1\,\text{mR/h}$

4. $\dfrac{I_1}{I_2} = \dfrac{(d_2)^2}{(d_1)^2}$

   $\dfrac{7}{I_2} = \dfrac{(2)^2}{(1)^2}$

   $\dfrac{7}{I_2} = \dfrac{4}{1}$ (cross-multiply)

   $4 I_2 = 7$
   $I_2 = 1.75\,\text{mR/h}$

5. $\dfrac{I_1}{I_2} = \dfrac{(d_2)^2}{(d_1)^2}$

   $\dfrac{6}{I_2} = \dfrac{(12)^2}{(6)^2}$

   $\dfrac{6}{I_2} = \dfrac{144}{36}$ (cross-multiply)

   $144 I_2 = 216$
   $I_2 = 1.5\,\text{mR/h}$

6. $\dfrac{I_1}{I_2} = \dfrac{(d_2)^2}{(d_1)^2}$

   $\dfrac{6}{I_2} = \dfrac{(6)^2}{(2)^2}$

   $\dfrac{6}{I_2} = \dfrac{36}{24}$ (cross-multiply)

   $36 I_2 = 24$
   $I_2 = 0.666\,\text{mR/h}$

7. $(10/5)^2$ $\quad 10 \div 5 = 2 \quad 2 \times 2 = 4$
8. $(12/4)^2$ $\quad 12 \div 4 = 3 \quad 3 \times 3 = 9$
9. $(4/1)^2$ $\quad 4 \div 1 = 4 \quad 4 \times 4 = 16$
10. $(8/2)^2$ $\quad 8 \div 2 = 4 \quad 4 \times 4 = 16$

Post-Test

1. Distance
2. declaration
3. The genetically significant dose (GSD) is the average annual gonadal equivalent dose to members of the population who are of childbearing age.
4. Scattered radiation
5. gonadal
6. "The intensity of radiation is inversely proportional to the square of the distance from the source."
7. restrain
8. Time, distance, and shielding
9. D
10. B
11. B
12. records
13. thickness
14. scattered

15.
$$\frac{I_1}{I_2} = \frac{(d_2)^2}{(d_1)^2}$$

$$\frac{10}{I_2} = \frac{(6)^2}{(3)^2}$$

$$\frac{10}{I_2} = \frac{36}{9} \text{ (cross-multiply)}$$

$$36 I_2 = 90$$
$$I_2 = 2.5 \text{ mR/h}$$

16. Secondary protective barrier
17. patient
18. 500 mSv (50 rem)
19. radiographer
20. 0.5, 0.05

Chapter 13

Exercise 1: Crossword Puzzle

Across: SYMPTOMS, PROSTATE, CONTAMINATED, POSITRON, DUST, ORIGIN, METABOLIC, PERIODIC, GEIGER, EXTERNAL, THYROID, SAFETY

Exercise 2: Matching

1. S	6. T	11. A	16. F	21. R
2. V	7. H	12. E	17. C	22. Q
3. K	8. O	13. Y	18. X	23. G
4. J	9. N	14. L	19. P	24. I
5. M	10. W	15. D	20. U	25. B

Exercise 3: Multiple Choice

1. C	6. D	11. C	16. D	21. C
2. C	7. A	12. B	17. B	22. C
3. D	8. C	13. D	18. C	23. C
4. C	9. B	14. B	19. D	24. D
5. C	10. A	15. C	20. B	25. C

Exercise 4: True or False

1. F (unstable)
2. T
3. T
4. F (unstable atom)
5. F (9 neutrons)
6. F (It is of concern to the general population.)
7. T
8. T
9. F (They are useful.)
10. F (short-lived radioisotopes)
11. F (No, technetium-99m is.)
12. T
13. T
14. T
15. F (Geiger counters)
16. F (Radiation therapy uses ionizing radiation for the treatment of disease, namely, cancer.)
17. T
18. F (A positron is a form of antimatter.)
19. T
20. T
21. F (These 511-keV photons cannot be shielded by an ordinary lead apron.)
22. T
23. T
24. T
25. T

Exercise 5: Fill in the Blank

1. 90, adjacent
2. metastases
3. 6, nucleus
4. Positron
5. prep
6. radiation
7. dirty bomb
8. radiosensitive
9. beta
10. electron capture
11. patient
12. unstable
13. annihilation
14. metabolic
15. Geiger
16. vary
17. plastic container
18. pregnant, 6
19. calcium
20. residual, sparing
21. isolated, minimize
22. radiotracer
23. 9
24. full
25. Monitoring

Exercise 6: Labeling
A.

Dose-Effect Relation After Acute Whole-Body Radiation from Gamma Rays or X-Rays*

Whole-Body Absorbed Dose	Effect
0.05 Gy	No symptoms
1. 0.15 Gy	No symptoms, but possible chromosomal aberrations in cultured peripheral-blood lymphocytes
2. 0.5 Gy	No symptoms (minor decreases in white-cell and platelet counts in a few persons)
3. 1 Gy	Nausea and vomiting in approximately 10% of patients within 48 hr after exposure
4. 2 Gy	Nausea and vomiting in approximately 50% of persons within 24 hr, with marked decreases in white-cell and platelet counts
5. 4 Gy	Nausea and vomiting in 90% of persons within 12 hr, and diarrhea in 10% within 8 hr; 50% mortality in the absence of medical treatment
6. 6 Gy	100% mortality within 30 days because of bone marrow failure in the absence of medical treatment
7. 10 Gy	Approximate dose that is survivable with the best medical therapy available
8. ≥10-30 Gy	Nausea and vomiting in all persons in less than 5 min; severe gastrointestinal damage; death likely in 2-3 wk in the absence of treatment
9. ≥30 Gy	Cardiovascular collapse and central nervous system damage, with death in 24-72 hr

*Gusev I, Guskova AK, Mettler FA Jr, eds: *Medical management of radiation accidents*, ed 2, Boca Raton, Fla, 2001, CRC Press.

Exercise 7: Short Answer

1. Therapeutic isotopes may be characterized by relatively long half-lives that are measured in terms of multiple days or multiple years and, with the exception of a few of them, usually quite high–energy radiation. The radiation may be in the form of gamma rays or fast electrons (beta radiation).
2. Electron capture occurs when an inner-shell electron is captured by one of the nuclear protons, followed directly by the two combining to produce a neutron.
3. In beta decay, a neutron transforms itself into a combination of a proton and an energetic electron (called a *beta particle*). There is also emission of another particle called a *neutrino*. The electron exits the nucleus and interacts with surrounding atoms. The decayed nucleus now has one additional proton, which results in a different element.
4. Diagnostic techniques in nuclear medicine typically make use of short-lived radioisotopes as radioactive tracers. These radionuclides have been attached to biologically active substances or chemicals, forming radioactive compounds that diffuse predominantly into certain regions or organs where scrutiny of particular physiologic processes is medically desired.
5. Positron emission tomography (PET) is an important imaging modality because it can examine metabolic processes within the body. This is particularly important with regard to the proliferation of cancer cells.
6. Fluorodeoxyglucose (FDG) is a radioactive tracer that not only is very similar in chemical behavior to ordinary glucose, and so will be taken up or metabolized by cancerous cells, but also will reveal their location through its positron emission decay and subsequent generation of oppositely traveling annihilation photons. These annihilation event sites are localizable through the PET scanner's ring of coincidence detectors.
7. If a PET scanner is physically joined in a tandem configuration with a CAT scanner to produce a single joint imaging device then, in essence, a facility gains the ability not only to detect the presence of abnormally high regions of glucose metabolism, yielding evidence that there is cancer spread, or metastasis, into other body areas, but also, at the same time, the means to obtain detailed information about the location and size of these lesions or growths.
8. After the attack on the World Trade Center on September 11, 2001, the possible use of other terrorist weapons, such as radiation, became a public health concern.
9. The Environmental Protection Agency (EPA) sets limits for radioactive contamination that assume that a 1-in-10,000 risk of causing a fatal cancer is unacceptable. This type of regulation requires hospitals, educational facilities, and industries to control accidental exposures so that the health of the population cannot be measurably affected. It also assumes that there are many other carcinogens present and that all are regulated to a similarly low level.
10. Personnel should wear gowns, masks, and gloves when working with a patient who has surface radioactive contamination.
11. The health care facility's radiation safety officer.
12. Normal badge limits do not apply during a radiation emergency.
13. Medical management during the first 48 hours of ARS involves simply treating the symptoms (e.g., nausea and vomiting) and trying to prevent dehydration.
14. Annihilation radiation is initiated by the radioactive decay of the nucleus of an unstable isotope. It is radiation in the form of two oppositely moving, 511-keV photons generated as the result of mutual annihilation of matter and antimatter (i.e., an electron and a positron).
15. A radioactive dispersal device, or dirty bomb, is a radioactive source mixed with conventional explosives. When such a device explodes, it spreads radioactive material through a specific area, causing contamination and panic.

Exercise 8: General Discussion or Opinion Questions

The questions in this exercise are intended to allow students to express their knowledge and understanding of the subject matter covered in this chapter. Because the answers may vary, determination of an answer's acceptability is left to the discretion of the instructor.

Post-Test

1. EPA
2. A radioactive dispersal device, or dirty bomb, is a radioactive source mixed with conventional explosives. When it explodes, this device spreads radioactive material through a specific area, causing contamination and panic.
3. Therapeutic radioisotopes are characterized by their relatively long half-lives, which are measured in terms of multiple days or multiple years and, with the exception of a few of them, usually quite high–energy radiation. The radiation may be in the form of gamma rays or fast electrons (beta radiation).
4. B
5. neutrons
6. Rapidly
7. A neutrino is a particle that has almost negligible mass and no charge but carries away any excess energy from the nucleus of the atom.
8. After a dirty bomb explodes, externally contaminated individuals can be decontaminated by removal of contaminated clothing and immersion in a shower to cleanse the skin.
9. Annihilation radiation
10. 2, 200
11. FDG
12. short-lived
13. 250 mSv (25 rem)
14. Electron capture is a process in which an inner-shell electron is captured by one of the nuclear protons followed directly by the two combining to produce a neutron.
15. Positron emitters result in the production of high-energy radiation.
16. Geiger-Müller (GM) detector (Geiger counter)
17. Technetium-99m
18. Radiation emergency plan and trained personnel
19. high-energy
20. beta